My First Pre[g

white
LADDER

Important note

The information in this book is not intended as a substitute for medical advice. Neither the authors nor White Ladder can accept any responsibility for any injuries, damages or losses suffered as a result of following the information herein.

My First Pregnancy
This first edition published in 2019 by White Ladder Press, an imprint of Crimson Publishing Ltd, 21d Charles Street, Bath BA1 1HX

© Crimson Publishing Ltd, 2019

British Library Cataloguing in Publication Data
A catalogue record for this book is available from the British Library

ISBN 978 1 910336 56 4

Front cover image: Leonid & Anna Dedukh/Adobe Stock

Printed and bound in Malta by Gutenberg Press Ltd

Contents

Congratulations!

You're pregnant! Welcome to one of the most amazing times of your life. Emotions may well be running high right now, and this book is here to hold your hand through this exciting new chapter.

Finding out you're pregnant can be the happiest and most magical time – it can also feel pretty daunting and scary. *My First Pregnancy* is written by a team of experts, giving you the latest medical advice to help you feel informed and in control of your pregnancy.

Pregnancy can often be downright uncomfortable and brings with it some unexpected side effects as your baby grows inside of you. We talk you through what you can expect to feel physically and emotionally, as well as the amazing development milestones your baby makes through each trimester.

Our team of experts includes Obstetric Consultant and Gynaecologist Dr Joanna Girling, midwife Pippa Nightingale, nutritionist Rana Conway, Pilates instructor Anya Hayes and parenting journalist Kate Street. Our experts share with you their wisdom in 'Words from the professionals', which you'll find throughout the book.

For ease of reading, we have referred to the baby as a boy throughout; midwives as female and doctors as male. For the same reason, we also assume your partner is male, however, advice given is usually equally relevant for same-sex couples.

From burgeoning bumps to birth plans and budgeting, *My First Pregnancy* includes everything you need to have a healthy and enjoyable pregnancy.

1

I'm pregnant!
Now what?

Whether this is a planned pregnancy or a surprise, this chapter will help you to deal with all the wild and wonderful thoughts that are rushing through your head. We'll cover what to do when you find out you are pregnant and how to prepare yourself for what happens next.

CONFIRMING YOU ARE PREGNANT

Whether you've been trying to get pregnant, or even if you just have your suspicions, confirming you are pregnant is the first important step you need to take. So what are some of the signs that you are pregnant?

These are some common first signs of pregnancy:

- an increased sense of taste or smell
- tender, bigger or 'tingling' breasts.
- feeling tired
- needing to pass urine more often
- an aversion to certain foods or drinks, or a craving for certain foods or drinks
- nausea
- feeling more emotional than normal.

For most women, though, the first sign that they might be pregnant is a missed period. If you find yourself thinking you might be pregnant, then you should try to have it confirmed as soon as possible so you can start looking after yourself (although ideally you are already in perfect health before you conceive!).

Pregnancy tests

When you become pregnant, the embryo (and later the placenta) produces a pregnancy hormone called human chorionic gonadotrophin (HCG). It plays a vital role in your baby's development, as it causes the follicle in the ovary from which the egg was released to produce the hormone progesterone, which itself prepares the lining of the uterus to feed the embryo and also causes the cessation of periods. The levels of HCG can be measured in your blood and urine. Most home pregnancy kits measure the level of this hormone in a sample of your urine and usually recommend that you take the test on or after the day your period is due.

Some new tests claim to give you a result five days *before* your due period, but the problem with this is that even people with regular periods can't be absolutely certain when conception and implantation occurred, and testing too early might lead to a false negative result.

 Words from the professionals

The best time to do the test is first thing in the morning when your urine is more concentrated, as (relatively speaking) there will be more of the hormone present in your urine if you are pregnant.

If you take a home pregnancy test and the indicator is very faint, wait a couple of days and test again, as it's possible that the embryo isn't generating sufficient amounts of HCG to register properly.

If you are undergoing fertility treatment it is advisable to wait up to 14 days after treatment before you take a pregnancy test because the hormones used can give you a false positive if the test is done early. Your IVF clinic will tell you when to perform the test.

Where should I take the test?

Most people choose to buy a home testing kit and see those results before going to the doctor. Home testing has advantages because your partner can be with you and you can do it at a time to suit you. However, if you prefer, you can have your first test done for free at your GP, family planning clinic or pharmacy.

If you do a test and the thin blue (or pink) line appears, then warm congratulations are in order – chances are you really are pregnant.

If you have good reason to suspect you are pregnant but have had a couple of negative pregnancy tests, it's probably a good idea to talk to your GP to see if a blood test might help to give you a definite answer.

I'M REALLY PREGNANT!

Even if you've been trying for a baby, discovering you are pregnant can still be a shock and it's totally normal to feel a range of emotions, from intense excitement to panic or fear. If the pregnancy wasn't planned, you might need longer to adjust to the news. Whatever your personal circumstances, give yourself a little time and space to get used to the idea.

Do I need to buy anything yet?

Hold off on buying the cot or booties for now, as it's more important that you start taking care of your health and wellbeing. Ideally you should already be taking 400 micrograms of folic acid daily, but if you're not, go to your local chemist or supermarket and buy some straightaway, as it can reduce the risk of having a baby born with a spinal cord defect such as spina bifida by up to 70%. There is some evidence to suggest that taking folic acid supplements also lowers the risk of having a baby born with a cleft lip or palate as well as lowering the chance of going into premature labour. And the most recent research from Holland suggests folic acid reduces the chance of the baby having a congenital heart defect by 20%.

If you haven't done so already, contact your GP surgery or local maternity unit directly to arrange your booking appointment (see page 10).

Start looking after yourself

The most important thing to do when you find out you are pregnant is to eat a healthy, well-balanced diet; stop smoking; avoid or reduce alcohol intake to no more than one or two units of alcohol once or twice a week; and take 400 micrograms of folic acid every day. It is also recommended that you take a supplement of 10 micrograms of Vitamin D (see page 100). If you have any health conditions or are on any medication you should discuss them with your GP as soon as you find out you are pregnant.

What should I be feeling?

There's no definitive answer to how you will be feeling in the very early stages of pregnancy: for some women, the hormones kick in very quickly and they experience strong symptoms almost as soon as the pregnancy is confirmed; other women can feel a bit anxious because they do not feel pregnant at all. Remember that every pregnancy is different and you'll have your own unique set of symptoms – lucky you!

In Chapter 2 we explore in detail all the changes you can expect over the coming 40 weeks but the symptoms you are most likely to experience in the early stages include the following.

- A missed period. Although this might sound somewhat obvious, some women do experience a light bleed, also known as spotting, at or shortly before the expected time of the period. This can occur after implantation, when the uterus lining is disturbed as the fertilised egg buries into it. This isn't necessarily anything to worry about, but if bleeding is painful, persistent, recurrent or occurs after your period was due, you should get it checked out by a health professional, in case you are having an ectopic pregnancy (see page 29).

- Nausea. Around half of all pregnant women experience some form of nausea or vomiting, with symptoms beginning around six weeks after their last period. Some women experience 'morning sickness' in the morning but it can happen at any time of the day, and some women find they begin experiencing nausea almost immediately.

- Needing to pee more often, especially at night.

- Exhaustion.

- A strange 'metallic' taste in the mouth.

- Going off certain foods or drink. Some people can't stand the taste of coffee or alcohol once they are pregnant, and one of the theories is that it is your body cleverly rejecting food or drink that isn't good for the growing baby.

- A heightened sense of smell.

- Tender, tingling or swollen breasts and darkening of the areola (the skin around the nipple).

- Increased vaginal discharge. This is normal as long as it is not associated with itchiness or soreness. If it is you should see your GP or midwife.

- Feling weepy or emotional.

- Being hungry all the time (despite the nausea).

More than one

Around one pregnancy in 65 will result in twins in the UK; it is very rare to have triplets or more. The majority (two-thirds) of twins are non-identical. Non-identical twins occur when you release more than one egg at ovulation, and both are fertilised by separate sperm. The babies may be of the same sex or different sex, and they will look no more alike than other brothers and sisters.

Identical twins account for about one-third of all twin pregnancies. Identical twins come about when one egg is fertilised by one sperm and then splits into two embryos shortly after conception. When this happens the twins will be of the same sex and have the same genes.

Twins are more likely if:

- you are an 'older' mother (late 30s or over)
- you have non-identical twins in your family
- you are taller and heavier than average
- you conceived using treatments such as IVF
- you are from Africa or Asia.

When carrying twins, you may experience heightened symptoms due to the additional HCG levels in your body, but this does not always happen. A multiple pregnancy is often confirmed at your first scan, and can be a shock when you've just got your head around the idea of having one baby! You will receive additional antenatal appointments and scans, especially towards the end. You may find that you need to reconsider some of your birth plan.

WORKING OUT YOUR DELIVERY DATE

The vast majority of babies are born between 37 and 42 weeks from the beginning of your last period. The EDD (estimated delivery date) is 40 weeks, but only 5% of babies arrive on that day; 90% of babies are born from three weeks before the due date to two weeks after – it might be better to have an EDM (estimated delivery month)!

As the average pregnancy lasts 266 days, you can count from the date of your last menstrual period and add 40 weeks – the two weeks before ovulation count as the first two weeks of pregnancy, even though you haven't even conceived at that point! Or, use Naegele's rule – add seven days to the first day of the last period and then take away three months. So, if your period started on 18 April, the EDD is 25 January.

If your cycle is regular but lasts less than 28 days you will need to subtract the number of days that it is less than 28 from your EDD; if it is longer than 28 days you will need to add the difference.

Once you see your doctor or midwife they will provide you an estimated date, but you will need to wait for an ultrasound to confirm this. Latest ultrasound guidance is that all EDDs should be based on scan measurements of the baby.

So be prepared for your due date to be adjusted. IVF pregnancies are excluded from this.

WHO AND WHEN TO TELL

Telling your loved ones is one of the most exciting parts of your early pregnancy. It is, however, something to consider carefully – many women choose to keep it among their nearest and dearest until the official dating scan (see page 17). This is when the greatest risk of miscarriage has passed, and you will feel confident sharing the good news. However, it's important to remember that should the unthinkable happen, you will also need support so may choose to tell those you feel confident in confiding in as soon as you take a positive test.

Telling your partner

If you are in a stable relationship, you will want to share the news with your partner as soon as possible if you were alone when you took the test. Enjoy this special moment!

If your pregnancy was unplanned or if you're not in a stable relationship, you might be feeling more anxious about sharing your news and what the future holds. It's up to you who you tell and when, but the best thing you can do is get support from people you trust and who can be there for you.

Telling your family

Many women want to share the news with their family straightaway; there's nothing nicer than telling your own mother that you're going to make her a granny. As mentioned, you might decide to hold off on spreading the news, but if there are problems in the pregnancy it may be that you will need their support. It's up to you whether you tell your entire family, just the prospective grandparents, or keep it a secret as a couple for a while.

Telling your friends

You may choose to tell your best friend straight away, while keeping it a secret from your wider group a little longer. Sometimes this is one of the hardest secrets to disguise, particularly if your friendships are regularly sealed by a large glass of wine on a Friday night. Many women hate lying to their mates, but if you are worried about telling them for whatever reason, the following excuses have come in handy.

- 'I'm on antibiotics' can be good, especially if you follow up with:
- 'I'm on those awful Flagyl tablets', because you *really* can't drink on those and by quoting the brand it makes the whole thing more plausible.

- 'I'm doing that seven-day detox.' If you are normally the 'health freak' of your social group the idea of you abstaining for a week might not be too surprising.
- Are you the gym bunny of your social circle? Then an impending marathon might buy you a few weeks of non-drinking time.
- Try telling just one close friend and see if they'll 'drink for two' and drink both your drinks! A tip if you go down this route – pick a mate with a good constitution who isn't planning on driving home!
- 'I'm driving.' An oldie but goodie, as no one can argue with you.

Some women also find telling certain friends can be difficult. There are those who might not seem overly thrilled as they realise that this will change your friendship forever, or there can be the awkwardness of telling those friends who you know have been trying for a baby of their own. The best thing you can do is be honest and ask people how they're feeling. If you understand where they're coming from it can help you to understand a perhaps less-than-perfect reaction.

Telling your work

We cover all the legal and practical aspects of your working pregnancy in Chapter 5, but officially you don't have to tell your employers until you are 25 weeks pregnant. By that time they might have guessed! It's probably not a bad idea to keep quiet until you have got through the first trimester of your pregnancy – unless you are experiencing such obvious pregnancy symptoms that they can't fail to notice or you need to take time off.

HOW YOU MIGHT BE FEELING

Your conception might have been planned with military precision or you may be one of the 40% of women whose pregnancy was unexpected. You may be giddy with excitement, and still struggling to get your head around it all. You might also have mixed feelings; don't feel bad if you are not as ecstatic or excited as you think you should be. Having a baby is undoubtedly a life-changing experience, and it's completely normal to have feelings of anxiety about the health of your growing baby, the delivery, and how it will impact on your life and relationships.

If you are experiencing a range of emotions about your pregnancy, remember your partner will probably be feeling the same. This is a perfect time to share all your hopes and fears together so that you can deal with anything that pregnancy might throw at you.

If the baby wasn't planned, you might have practical considerations to take into account, like the stability of your relationship, your finances or maybe your career.

With pregnancy hormones raging around their bodies it's little wonder that many newly pregnant women find themselves inexplicably in tears over the smallest things. If you're feeling overwhelmed by the news, just take it a day at a time and remember that women have been having babies for thousands of years without scans, epidurals, or even doctors around. It really is the most natural thing in the world!

What you might be worrying about

All of your fears are normal and natural. Here are a few common concerns and some advice to help you calm your fears.

'I got drunk before I knew I was pregnant.'

This is a very common worry, as a glass (or three) of your favourite tipple is often what gets us in the mood for baby-making in the first place. Try not to worry if you did overindulge because a one-off boozy session is unlikely to have done any damage to the fetus, although it may increase the chance of miscarriage. Try not to beat yourself up about it, but once you have confirmed that you are pregnant it is advisable to cut out regular drinking. An occasional glass is unlikely to harm your baby but you should always read up on the latest medical advice. See page 85 for more information on drinking and pregnancy.

'I went to a music festival, got stoned and found out a week later I was expecting.'

There is clear evidence to show that taking recreational drugs during pregnancy can pose a risk to your baby's health and development, so even if you are only an occasional recreational user it is strongly advised that you stop before you conceive or once you discover you are pregnant. If you did take drugs before you found out, you should discuss it with your midwife or obstetrician.

'I smoked two packets of fags on a girls' night out.'

If you or your partner are a smoker it's time to stub out your habit, because studies have shown that smoking (and passive smoking) is detrimental to the unborn child. Smoking slows down the growth of the baby, reduces the baby's brain development, makes premature delivery more likely, and increases the chance of cot death (sudden infant death syndrome) after the birth. Recent evidence from Scotland suggests it may increase the chance of an ectopic pregnancy.

It is really important that both you and your partner try to stop together, as this will help your determination and reduces the effects of passive smoking. Try nicotine replacement gums and patches, e-cigarettes or access the NHS Stop Smoking counselling service – your midwife or GP should be able to direct you to them. Smoking also increases the chance of getting thrombosis (blood clots) in your legs or lungs, so that is another reason to stop. Always talk openly with your midwife and GP and seek their advice and support. A lot of people struggle to give up smoking, so do ask for the guidance you need to help you through. You are four times more likely to quit smoking if you seek help. Look at www.nhs.uk/smokefree.

'I'm addicted to …'

It's easy to advise you to stop all your guilty pleasures when you are pregnant, but you may be addicted to nicotine, alcohol or drugs and even though you know you should give up for the sake of your baby, you can't. If you do have an addiction and find out you are pregnant, go to your GP straightaway to seek help and advice.

'I'm really overweight; how will I manage when I'm pregnant?'

Although you may think that being pregnant is the best excuse ever to put on weight, you'll soon find that you shouldn't gain as much weight as you might think and that you need to monitor your diet carefully. Being seriously overweight while pregnant can cause problems such as miscarriage, diabetes in pregnancy, thrombosis and pre-eclampsia (see page 64).

You should talk with your doctor about taking a higher dose of folic acid. Your doctor or midwife will advise you on how to maintain/start a healthy eating and exercise regime during your pregnancy, and will usually recommend that you gain as little weight as possible.

ANTENATAL CARE

Antenatal care is designed to help make sure you and your baby are both as healthy as possible during pregnancy and delivery. Even if you are healthy, you still need careful check-ups as the extra burden of pregnancy can occasionally cause or reveal problems. If you already have some health or lifestyle issues, then antenatal care will help support you and your baby.

Your antenatal care options may include:

- shared care between your GP and a midwife

- midwife- or GP-led care

- hospital-based consultant-led care if your pregnancy is likely to need extra monitoring for you or the baby

- private independent midwife for antenatal care and delivery

- private maternity care with an obstetrician/midwife. The whole package can cost around £5,000–£10,000.

Some women have a nominated midwife they will see at every appointment and hopefully at the birth too; other women will see a different midwife each time they visit – some health authorities run what's called a 'Domino Scheme', where a team of community midwives look after you. Systems vary depending on where you live and your antenatal care will also depend on the type of birth you are planning. If you have any chronic health conditions such as diabetes, epilepsy, high blood pressure or inflammatory bowel disease, ideally you will be able to see your GP, obstetrician or hospital doctor to discuss the issues relevant to the pregnancy before you conceive, and plan the antenatal care you will need. Similarly, if you take any medication you should talk to your GP, obstetrician or hospital doctor. If you are at increased risk of delivering early, your hospital may offer you an appointment at the Pre-term Birth Clinic. If you have serious mental health problems you may be referred to a Perinatal Mental Health Team.

Thinking about your options

Before you go to the doctor it is useful to have some idea about where you would like to give birth, as this will help to ensure you are booked into the right kind of hospital for you. A really useful website to help you with this is www.which.co.uk/birth-choice. It takes you through all of your birth options and has a really helpful section with statistics about maternity units in your local area, so you can make informed choices about where you want your baby to be born and have some ideas about the care you might like to receive.

Your birthing options may include:

- NHS consultant-led hospital maternity unit
- NHS midwife-led birth centre – freestanding or alongside a hospital
- home birth
- private maternity unit attached to an NHS hospital
- private hospital that exclusively deals with maternal and child health.

The pros and cons of each are outlined in detail in Chapter 7. Some hospitals are in such demand they get booked up very quickly. If you pick a hospital that is not local, bear in mind that you might go into labour during rush hour and a trip across town in heavy traffic might not be the best idea! Also, postnatal midwifery is organised by the hospital in whose catchment your address falls, not the one where you delivered, so you could miss out on continuity of care.

YOUR BOOKING APPOINTMENT

If you know which hospital you wish to deliver in, check their website as you may be able to make a 'self-referral'. If you can't self-refer, or you don't know where to book, make an appointment with your GP as soon as you can. The booking appointment may take place at the hospital, a clinic, maternity unit, GP surgery or at home.

What is a booking appointment?

It is believed that the term 'booking' originates from a time when women literally had to 'book' their hospital bed for labour. (In some parts of the country it could be argued that the same applies now.)

It's your first official check-up during your pregnancy, and should provide the team looking after you with valuable background information about your health that may have an impact on your baby.

It is recommended that you have your booking appointment no later than week 10 of your pregnancy: the reason for this is that you might need some tests that should be done in the first trimester of pregnancy (ie by 13 weeks) and they are organised once you have completed your initial consultation.

What to expect at your first appointment

Questions, questions and more questions … at the end of it you might feel that applying for a job at NASA would be an easier option, but don't worry: none of the other antenatal appointments is as detailed as this one. Some of the questions will relate to the father, so it is ideal if he attends too. What questions will the midwife ask?

- **The date of the first day of your last period.** This is so your due date can be estimated and allows the midwife to book the dating scan at the right time; this gives an accurate picture (literally) of how pregnant you are and how many babies you've made. There are more details on antenatal scans on page 17.

- **Your obstetric history.** Details of any previous pregnancies, including terminations, miscarriages and stillbirths. This helps to plan the type of care you will need.

- **Your general health.** This includes any significant medical problems, especially those that require you to take medication or visit a doctor regularly. The pregnancy might influence the medical condition (often improving it!) and the medical condition might influence the pregnancy (for example, women with high blood pressure are more likely to develop pre-eclampsia, see page 64). Your midwife will also assess the chance of you having a thrombosis in pregnancy (see page 64). If you suffer from asthma, you have a higher chance of giving birth early, evidence suggests. Tell your doctor and make sure you are monitored appropriately.

- **Your (and your partner's) family history of genetic conditions.** You can now screen the baby for certain genetic conditions like cystic fibrosis or sickle cell disease, which the midwife will organise for you if appropriate.

Words from the professionals

NICE (the National Institute for Health and Care Excellence) now recommends that women at higher risk of developing pre-eclampsia are offered a low dose of aspirin from 12 weeks.

- **Your (and your partner's) family history of illnesses.** These include heart disease and diabetes, among others.

- **Your mental health.** If you are prone to depression or have ever had any mental health problems, it is important that you make the midwife aware of this because you may need extra help or support during pregnancy or after the birth. There are some mental health issues that have high chances of recurring after delivery, so treatment to prevent this may be considered. If your mother or a sister has had a serious postnatal mental health problem, you should tell your midwife.

 Words from the professionals

At least one in 10 women have some form of mental health problems, and many units have specialised midwives to give extra support or direct you to appropriate counselling or psychiatric services.

- **Your lifestyle.** The midwife will want to find out how many units of alcohol you drink and whether or not you smoke cigarettes or use recreational drugs. She might give you advice about how both can affect your developing baby, and point you towards services that help you quit if you are having trouble.

- **Domestic violence.** There is evidence that domestic violence gets worse in pregnancy, and up to nine in 100 women are affected during or shortly after pregnancy. So, now all women are asked about domestic violence – this is your opportunity to speak up in a safe and protective environment. If you need help in this area, call the freephone 24-hour National Domestic Violence helpline on 0808 2000 247.

- **Your sexual health.** Chlamydia is increasingly common in young women, and if you are under 25 you might receive information on screening for this as the disease can be passed on to the unborn child.

- **Your smear history.** If you are over 25 you should have a cervical smear every three years to test for signs that could lead to cervical cancer. While routine smears are not usually performed in pregnancy, a repeat smear after a previously abnormal one should be done in pregnancy. If you have had treatment to your cervix after an abnormal smear you may be at increased risk of premature delivery and may need extra care.

- **Your preferences regarding delivery.** If you haven't decided where to have the baby, the midwife will go through all the birth options available to you in your locality. It's really important that you ask lots of questions about the type of care on offer because it may affect where and how you give birth. Ask if you will see the same midwife each time, if that's important to you, or whether you need to see a consultant.

- **About FGM (Female Genital Mutilation).** Many women from North Africa, some parts of the Middle East and Asia have had FGM performed on them in childhood. It is important for the team looking after you to know this, so they can help you and your daughters (it is illegal to do or allow FGM on a UK-born female).

If you are in a same-sex relationship, it is a good idea to ask the midwife to put a note on your maternity notes, explaining briefly about your family. This will inform any future healthcare provider and you won't feel the pressure to explain yourself at every appointment or scan.

What will the midwife do?

Blood tests

If you are worried about needles, take your partner or a friend to distract you, as you will need to give a sample of blood.

You will be tested for syphilis, HIV and hepatitis B – if you have any of these you will be offered treatment for yourself and to reduce the chance of your baby becoming infected too. You will be checked for anaemia (usually caused by low iron levels) and for sickle cell disease and thalassaemia. These are inherited forms of anaemia that are mostly very mild, but if you or your partner both have a mild form (or 'trait') you could have a baby with a more serious form of the illness.

You will get to know your blood group – this means that if you need a blood transfusion, the right blood can be prepared more quickly. If you have a religious or other objection to blood transfusions it is important that you discuss this with your midwife early in the pregnancy. If your blood group is Rhesus (Rh) negative you will be offered an injection at around 28 weeks.

Blood pressure

The midwife will take your blood pressure at every antenatal appointment. The first reading will act as a baseline for future checks and will also allow her to tell if your blood pressure is already high – if it is she will probably ask you to see an obstetrician. Usually your blood pressure is lower in pregnancy than before you conceive.

Words from the professionals

If a Rhesus negative woman is pregnant with a Rhesus positive baby, and if the baby's blood crosses the placenta into the mother's blood, the mother can develop antibodies against Rhesus positive blood – and these antibodies can make the baby anaemic, sometimes dangerously so. The Anti D injection, given at around 28 weeks, helps to stop this from happening. More and more hospitals are offering a blood test at 16 weeks to Rhesus negative women to check their baby's Rhesus group – only women carrying a baby predicted to be Rhesus positive need Anti D injections.

A rise in blood pressure in the second half of your pregnancy might indicate that you are developing pre-eclampsia (see page 64), which can be dangerous to you and your baby.

Carbon monoxide testing

Women who smoke have higher Carbon monoxide (CO) levels than women not exposed to cigarette fumes. CO is a poisonous gas that can build up in your blood, replacing oxygen and reducing the amount of oxygen you and the baby receive. If you are a smoker, your midwife might offer to do a breath test to measure the level in your body – this is usually with a hand-held machine that you blow into and which gives an immediate reading. More than 3 COppm (molecules of CO per million parts of air) is considered high enough to warrant offering further smoking cessation support. Some women find this test a useful way to see how their CO levels fall as they manage to cut down, and it can be really motivating (see page 88).

Urine testing

You will need to produce a fresh urine sample at every appointment. She will dip a chemical strip into it to check for signs of a urine infection. If an infection is suspected, the sample will be sent to the laboratory where it will be possible to make a definite diagnosis. Urine infections are much more common in pregnancy, and are treated with antibiotics to decrease the chance of getting a kidney infection (or that you will go into premature labour).

In the second half of your pregnancy the midwife will also be looking for protein, since this can be another sign of pre-eclampsia (or a sign of urine infection, vaginal discharge, or not catching the sample cleanly). Recent advice from NICE advises using an automated urine stick reader for protein, so you may see your sample going into a machine!

Weights and measures

Your weight and height will be recorded at this first appointment and your midwife will calculate your BMI (body mass index). This determines if you are underweight (BMI less than 19), normal (BMI 19–25), overweight (BMI 25–30) or obese (BMI more than 30).

If your BMI is between 19 and 30 you probably will not be weighed again. If it is over 30, you may need to see a doctor to look into why this might be and what extra care you might need, as you are more likely to have pregnancy complications. If you are underweight you may also need to see a doctor to explore why this is. For more information on weight gain during pregnancy see page 102.

Your antenatal notes

You might be given your antenatal notes at the end of your booking appointment or they might be given to you when the blood results are in. You should keep them with you at all times – unfortunately you never know when you might feel unwell or have an accident, and you must always show them to any healthcare professional looking after you so that they understand your pregnancy. You must bring them to each appointment you have during your pregnancy.

If you go on holiday, particularly towards the end of your pregnancy, it's important to take them with you in case you go into labour early or have an urgent medical problem and need to visit a doctor or a hospital.

Initially the notes will contain much of what you have told the midwife on that first antenatal visit, such as your name, address and hospital number; ethnic group and religion; past and present illnesses; current treatment/medicines taken, etc.

The midwife will also record test results, or you will be given computer-generated reports and scan details such as the size of your baby's head and length of his femur. As your pregnancy progresses, the measurement of your bump, the position of the baby, and the baby's heartbeat will also be recorded. Pregnancy problems/complications or additional unscheduled visits to the antenatal clinic will be also be noted. There will probably be a birth plan section where your preferences regarding labour and birth can be completed but you don't have to do this right now. You're quite likely to change your mind by the time the baby arrives and it's probably a good idea to give yourself time to read up and discuss all the options available to you. Practical information such as phone numbers for your GP, midwife, NHS Direct, the hospital switchboard and delivery ward will also be included.

Your notes will also contain advice on what to do in a potential emergency situation in pregnancy.

Deciphering your notes

These are some of the most common abbreviations you might find in your notes:

GA (gestational age or pregnancy duration). If it says you are 10+2 it means you are 10 weeks and two days pregnant (counting from your period, not from when you actually conceived).

Urine. NAD indicates nothing abnormal detected.

BP. Ideal blood pressure is less than 140/90, and generally the lower the better. If either figure is higher you will probably need extra monitoring to see if pre-eclampsia is developing; if either the upper figure is more than 140, or the lower one more than 90, you may need treatment.

Height of your uterus. Once your pregnancy is well underway, your midwife will be measuring the height of your uterus. Also known as fundal height, this measurement is taken from the top of your bump to the top of your pubic bone, and the length in centimetres should roughly correspond to the number of weeks pregnant you are: = D or = dates means you are measuring the correct size for your pregnancy dates. The main aim is to pick up if the baby seems too small.

FH (fetal heart). The midwife will either record the number of beats per minute of your baby's heart, or write the abbreviation FHH, meaning fetal heart heard.

FM (fetal movements). This refers to whether you or the midwife have felt the baby move.

Baby's position. Towards the end of your pregnancy the midwife will record your baby's position, using the following abbreviations:

- Ceph = cephalic. This means the baby is head down and in position for birth.
- Br = breech. This means the baby is bottom down.
- LOA = left occiput anterior. This means the back of the baby's head is on your left-hand side and towards the front of your stomach.
- LOP = left occiput posterior. This means the back of the baby's head is on your left, and towards your back.
- ROA = right occiput anterior. This means the baby's head is at the right side of your stomach at the front.
- ROP = right occiput posterior. This means the baby's head is on the right side of your stomach towards the back.

ANTENATAL APPOINTMENTS

Antenatal clinic appointments can be with your GP, a midwife, a hospital doctor or a mixture. They may take place in a community or children's centre, the GP surgery, the hospital or a mixture. After booking, there is usually a 'minimum schedule' of care. You will have around 10 clinic appointments at 16, 25, 28, 31, 34, 36, 38, 40, 41 and 42 weeks. However, this schedule will depend on how well you and the baby are, whether you are having twins and what type of care you have chosen/been offered.

At each visit your blood pressure and urine will be checked, your tummy examined, usually the baby's heart listened to, and your questions answered. The whole point of the appointments is to make sure you and the baby are both well, and to investigate any concerns detected.

After about 26 weeks of pregnancy, you will usually have your bump measured at each visit. Traditionally this measurement in centimetres agrees with the number of weeks of pregnancy. However this doesn't allow for your size, or your age or ethnic origin. Because of this, some units have recently started to use customised charts which do allow for your age, BMI and ethnicity. The inventors of these charts claim that they allow better detection of babies who are smaller than they are meant to be – and this is important because they might be at increased risk of stillbirth (see page 30). Always keep a close eye on your baby's movements and tell your midwife or maternity unit the same day if they slow down. Make sure you attend all your appointments – they are really worthwhile!

ANTENATAL SCANS

According to guidelines from NICE women should be offered two routine ultrasound scans during pregnancy: a dating scan at around 10–14 weeks and an anomaly scan at around 18–22 weeks. However, if you have pain or bleeding you may need an earlier scan. There is no evidence that extra scans or 3D or 4D scans help in a normal pregnancy.

Until you have the first scan it is sometimes difficult to believe that you really are having a baby – even if you are throwing up every 10 minutes! The scan makes the whole thing very real. When you go for your scans it is advisable to bring someone with you if you can, as there is a possibility that the sonographer might pick up a problem and if that happens it's better to have someone to support you. About 3% of babies have structural problems, many of which can be detected by the scan. Sometimes a miscarriage is unexpectedly diagnosed at the scan.

Dating scan: 10–14 weeks

You will be seen by a sonographer: this is a radiographer or midwife or doctor who is specially trained to conduct ultrasound scans. You might be asked to attend the appointment with a full bladder, as this helps push up the uterus and give a clearer picture. Probably the most painful aspect of the whole process is sitting with your legs crossed in a packed waiting room with a bladder fit to explode. Drink about a pint of water an hour before your appointment.

When you go in, you'll be asked to pull your top up and your bottoms down and gel will be wiped across your bare tummy – it may be freezing, so be prepared. The sonographer will glide a probe across your stomach and an image of the fetus will appear on a small monitor beside you. Don't be frightened if they work in silence – it takes a huge amount of concentration to scan well. They look at the fetus from every angle, taking the vital measurements that will give an accurate picture of the 'date' of your growing baby. The crown–rump measurement is the most accurate way in the first trimester to determine the baby's age – from the top of his head to his bottom. Once they have all the essential information, they'll talk you through the image on the screen, and point out the baby's heart beating and different parts of the body. It is common for the baby's position to mean that not all structures can be seen at one visit – you might be asked to return for another scan in a few days or weeks.

The dating scan isn't just to give you an idea of when your baby is due: it also confirms how many babies you are carrying and can detect some severe structural problems in the baby. Sadly, the scan can also pick up the news that no expectant woman wants to hear: that the pregnancy is no longer viable and the baby has died or is unlikely to survive.

Most hospitals will give you a print-out of an image of your baby at this scan for a nominal charge. Buy at least two copies: one can go into your newborn's memory box and the second can live in your wallet to be whipped out at every opportunity. Mostly the photos are similar to Polaroids and will fade – so take more permanent copies if you can.

Transvaginal scan

If you are overweight, your uterus is in a certain position or if the length of your cervix needs to be measured, the sonographer might suggest a transvaginal scan. If this happens they will gently insert a transducer – a thin probe – into your vagina. It doesn't hurt and won't harm you or the baby, so don't panic if you have to have one: it's about as uncomfortable as inserting a tampon and does give a much clearer picture.

Nuchal translucency (NT) scan

The nuchal translucency scan is when the sonographer measures the collection of fluid within the skin at the back of your baby's neck (all babies have some fluid present). It is performed between 11 and 14 weeks (often alongside the dating scan), and there is strong evidence to suggest that if there is a deeper accumulation of fluid present there is an increased chance of your baby having Down's syndrome. The sonographer may also look to see if the baby's nasal bone is visible: if it is not, this is another marker indicating a chance of Down's. However, not all medical professionals agree that examining the nasal bone is helpful, so it is not widely done. This scan can be performed along with a blood test, testing for hormone levels in the maternal blood. When this is done, it is called the combined screening test, and is available to everyone free of charge on the NHS (see page 22).

Fetal anomaly scan: 18–22 weeks

Around this time in your pregnancy you will be booked in for your second scan: the fetal anomaly scan. This looks for anomalies (things that differ from the norm) in your growing baby. The procedure is very similar to the dating scan, except that the scan takes much longer because the sonographer has many more things to look at now that your baby has grown. There are some abnormalities that will be very apparent at this scan and some that cannot be detected until after birth, so you must be aware that, even if you are told everything appears normal, this is no guarantee of your baby being born without any health problems (autism or cerebral palsy, for example, cannot be seen on scans).

The scan will also measure the size of your baby's head (head circumference), waist (abdominal circumference) and leg (femur length), and these measurements are plotted on a chart showing their size in relation to other babies of the same gestational age. This allows final confirmation of your EDD. Occasionally if the baby is unusually small, extra tests may be offered to see if there may be a problem causing this.

The scan also measures the amniotic fluid, referred to on the scan report usually as AFI (amniotic fluid index). This fluid is made by the baby's kidneys (ie it is his urine) and the placenta, and circulates through the baby as he swallows it and then pees it! Too much or too little may indicate or cause a problem.

It's not just the baby the sonographer will be looking at: the position of the placenta will be noted, in case it causes difficulties later on (see box below) and you may be asked to come back to be scanned nearer your due date if

Low-lying placenta or placenta praevia

The placenta is the organ that acts as a life support system to your fetus. It is the conduit which passes oxygen and nutrition from mother to baby.

Sometimes, though, the placenta implants low in the uterus and covers – or nearly covers – the cervix (the entrance to the uterus). After 16 weeks of pregnancy this is called placenta praevia if it covers or partly covers the cervix, and low-lying if it is within 20mm of the cervix. In 90% of cases it moves out of the way before the baby is due but in 10% of cases it doesn't. This is a potentially risky condition, as it can cause severe maternal bleeding, and if it is blocking your baby's exit route you'll almost certainly need to have your baby by planned Caesarean section. See also page 27 for what might happen if the scan suggests your baby has a problem.

it is lower than expected. The placenta will be described as being anterior or posterior (ie at the front or back of the uterus) and either normal (ie away from the cervix), or low (ie lying within 20mm of the cervix), or praevia (partially or completely covering the cervix). You should be offered another scan at 32–36 weeks, depending on how low your placenta is.

If you do have placenta praevia you should have the opportunity to discuss this with a member of staff and be given an information leaflet. You may be advised not to travel, to abstain from sex and to take iron tablets. If you do experience any bleeding, you should get to the hospital straightaway.

Finally, if you have an increased chance of pre-term delivery, you may be offered a transvaginal scan to measure the length of your cervix.

Pink or blue?

The sex of the baby can often be detected at the anomaly scan, but do bear in mind it may not be the policy of your hospital to tell you. The sonographer's determination of the sex of your baby is also not 100% accurate, as the umbilical cord can be mistaken for a penis, and some Buddha babies like to cross their legs and make it difficult for the sonographer to see. In a recent study, sonographers could identify the sex of only 46% of babies at 13 weeks and 80% at 20 weeks. If you do want to know, it's advisable to tell the person scanning you at the outset so they have a chance to have a look in the time allotted for your appointment.

TESTING FOR DOWN'S SYNDROME

Down's syndrome is named after John Langdon Down, the doctor who first identified it. Down's syndrome is a genetic disorder that affects around one in 1,000 babies. We know that babies with Down's syndrome inherit an extra copy of the number 21 chromosome, but it's not known exactly why this occurs. When your egg is being prepared for release (and therefore for pregnancy) the chromosomes separate, so that instead of being in pairs (as they are in all cells apart from egg and sperm), they are single. At conception, the chromosomes in the sperm and those in the egg join together to form pairs again, meaning that the genes of the baby are a mixture of the mum and dad's. However, sometimes the chromosomes in the egg do not separate correctly and both of the chromosomes – in this case pair number 21 – join with the number 21 in the sperm, meaning that the baby has 47 chromosomes instead of the usual 46, resulting in Down's syndrome. It is also possible for the extra chromosome 21 to come from the sperm, but this is less common unless the man is over 60 years old.

Babies born with Down's syndrome will typically have a flat facial profile and the back of their head will be flat. Their eyes slant upwards, and they have smaller ears and a protruding tongue. They are likely to have floppy joints and poor muscle tone, and other problems may include impairment of their sight, hearing, heart or digestive system. Down's syndrome children tend to develop at a slower pace and are likely to have learning difficulties.

There is no cure for Down's syndrome but modern education and therapeutic services have progressed to the point where a Down's syndrome diagnosis is not the devastating blow it once was. Instead, people with this disability are able to integrate into society almost as easily as anyone else.

Chances of having a baby with Down's syndrome

We may not know exactly why Down's syndrome occurs but we do know that it increases with maternal age. A girl is born with all her eggs already inside her, meaning her eggs age as she does. Older eggs are less able to separate their chromosomes than younger ones, so the chance of having a baby with Down's syndrome increases proportionally to the mother's age. By way of illustration, consider that pregnant women aged 20 have a chance of one in 1,500 of having a baby with Down's syndrome, while a woman aged 30 has a chance of one in 900, and a 40-year-old woman has a chance of one in 100.

Should I take a test?

There are two stages to the process of testing for Down's: the first is a screening test, which indicates the *likelihood* of you carrying a Down's baby, and the second stage is a diagnostic test, which will give you a *definite* answer. All pregnant women who book before 20 weeks should be offered a test to screen their pregnancy for Down's syndrome. You do not have to have the test and you should consider your ethical, moral or religious position for and against testing. About 750,000 women are offered the Down's test annually and 60% take up the offer. Once you have decided if you want the test or not, just tell your midwife and she will ensure your wishes are complied with.

If you feel you might not be able to continue the pregnancy if your baby is given a diagnosis of Down's syndrome, or would like more time to adjust to the idea of having a baby with the condition, you should probably take the test. But remember that the screening test does not diagnose Down's syndrome – it only shows what the likelihood is: 3%–5% of all women will have a 'positive' screening test. For many of these women, the baby will not have Down's syndrome. If the test results show that your baby has an increased likelihood of Down's syndrome then you will be offered a diagnostic test.

Screening tests for Down's syndrome

There are several screening tests available. Which one you are offered will depend on whether you are less than 14 weeks pregnant or not and what your particular hospital has available.

Single blood test

Some health authorities will offer blood tests that show an increased chance of Down's through markers in the blood. They may measure two (double), three (triple) or even four (quadruple) substances – the more they measure, the more accurate the test. This test is done between 15 weeks and 20 weeks. The results of the test analysis, combined with the mother's age and the stage of the pregnancy, are fed into a computer and the result will give a statistical chance of Down's syndrome. If this is between one in two and one in 250 you will be offered a diagnostic test.

Combined test

Some hospitals will also perform an NT scan (see page 18), and combine the blood test results with the NT measurements to get an even more accurate assessment of risk; this is called a combined test, and is done between 11 weeks and 13 weeks plus six days. The latest figures reveal that the combined test detects between 75% and 90% of cases of Down's syndrome.

If you want a combined test and the NT scan isn't offered in your area, you can choose to visit one of the 100 private screening centres in the country. It costs between £100 and £200 depending on where you live. You can ask your midwife for details of local centres or call the Fetal Medicine Centre (see page 262) for a list of accredited centres.

Non-invasive prenatal testing (NIPT) using cell-free fetal DNA (CFF DNA)

This new blood test screening for Down's, Edwards' and Patau's syndromes will be offered to women with a 1 in 150 or higher chance on their first screening test and is expected to become available on the NHS during 2019 but a date has not been set yet. Until then the test is widely available privately. The test looks for traces of the baby's DNA in your blood. A small blood sample is taken from your arm, any time from 10 weeks of pregnancy, and the chance of your baby having Down's syndrome is estimated. While it may produce some false positives, these can be confirmed by follow-up diagnostic invasive testing. It is likely to widely reduce the number of women taking the invasive test. The downsides are the wait for a result (currently around two weeks) and that there isn't a guarantee you will get a result – estimates suggest a result for 95% of women.

Diagnostic tests

The RCOG (Royal College of Obstetricians and Gynaecologists) recently estimated that around 30,000 women are offered a diagnostic test each year in the UK, or 5% of all pregnant women. You will be offered either chorionic villus sampling (CVS) or an amniocentesis test. CVS can usually be performed between 11 and 14 weeks, whereas amniocentesis is carried out from 15 weeks.

Words from the professionals

There is an additional risk of miscarriage with amniocentesis of 1% and a 1%–2% additional chance of miscarriage with CVS, although the risk varies from hospital to hospital. Be aware. Recent research indicates that two healthy babies are miscarried, as a result of the diagnostic tests, for every three Down's syndrome babies detected, so it is important that you know the risks of having an invasive test.

In both procedures a fine needle is inserted into the uterus; this can be done vaginally for CVS or trans-abdominally for CVS and amniocentesis. Don't panic that your baby will be touched by the needle: an ultrasound probe will be guiding the doctor to ensure that he has a clear picture of the position of the needle and your baby.

Latest RCOG guidance also ensures that doctors only continue to do these tests if they have sufficient experience each year – set at 30 cases. Therefore, you may find that you are asked to go to another hospital for the test, since some units are combining their resources to ensure the best levels of experience for their doctors and fewer complications.

A sample of tissue from the placenta (the chorionic villi) will be removed if you undergo CVS and a sample of the amniotic fluid is extracted if you undergo amniocentesis. The actual test only takes a couple of minutes and you should have the results back within a few weeks. Many hospitals now offer rapid testing for chromosomes 13, 18 and 21, with results being available in three to five working days.

Regional variations

There is evidence to suggest that there is a postcode lottery when it comes to Down's syndrome screening. London hospitals currently have the highest detection rates, while the lowest detection rates are occurring in the North and Midlands areas of the UK.

If your local hospital relies on just a single blood test or NT scan you may consider having a more accurate test privately. In some hospitals up to a third of Down's syndrome babies are not detected before birth, whereas in other areas 20% of women go through needless diagnostic invasive tests that could risk them losing the baby (see below).

Regional variation in diagnosis of Down's reflects availability of tests, but also maternal factors – such as age of mother, social deprivation and cultural beliefs – influence uptake of tests.

Most women describe the procedure as uncomfortable as opposed to painful. CVS has been likened to having a smear test and amniocentesis can make your tummy a bit sore afterwards. Slight cramping and very mild vaginal bleeding afterwards are normal, although if you have heavy bleeding, clear vaginal fluid loss or flu-like symptoms you should seek immediate medical assistance.

For more information on Down's syndrome, visit www.downs-syndrome.org.uk. For more information on screening and diagnostic tests, visit www.arc-uk.org.

 Words from the professionals

Around 90% of women choose to terminate if they get a positive confirmation of Down's syndrome, but others choose to continue the pregnancy. If you have a high screening test result, you might want to opt for CVS (as opposed to amniocentesis) because it can be done earlier in your pregnancy.

GOING PRIVATE

Private scan options

We have outlined the routine evidence-based scans you can expect to receive on the NHS unless there is a potential problem with you or the baby that your midwife or consultant wants to keep an eye on. There are other scans available if you have the money to pay for them, but outside the NHS the standard setting and auditing of results may be different, and so the quality not so good. You also need to think through why you want a scan – and discuss it again with your doctor or midwife. Women commonly ask for a scan to reassure themselves that the baby is OK, but unfortunately the scan cannot do that. It is usually better to talk about what is worrying you, rather than pay large sums of money for a scan that may not be helpful.

Costs for private scans

The number and type of scans you can pay for vary widely from region to region. Below is an indication of what prices you would expect to pay:

- cost of a private appointment: £80 to £150
- cost of a nuchal translucency scan (2D Imaging) (11–14 weeks): £170 to £250
- cost of a soft markers/detailed fetal anatomy scan (2D Imaging) (16–22 weeks): £220 to £320
- cost of reassurance scans, including sexing (14–22 weeks): £100 to £180.

Unnecessary 'souvenir' pictures

There isn't any evidence to show that two or three scans will harm your baby, but having unnecessary scans to fill your family photo album may not be the best idea. According to the latest research from the Health Protection Agency (HPA), there can be risks associated with an unnecessarily large number of scans. If there isn't a medical reason for having a scan you might want to think twice about having one.

Private tests

Non-invasive prenatal testing (NIPT)

This test for Down's syndrome looks for traces of the baby's DNA in your blood. See page 21 for more information. It is not currently widely available on the NHS, but it should be soon. Private clinics offer the test for around £500, but the cost is falling and some centres charge less than £300.

Group B Streptococcus

Group B Streptococcus (Group B Strep or GBS) is a common bacterium that's carried in the vagina of around 25% of pregnant woman. It is usually harmless, but it can be passed from mother to baby during birth, and occasionally this causes very serious health problems in the baby.

Around 75 babies die annually from neonatal Group B Strep, and 40 sustain long-term health problems. If GBS is detected incidentally during other antenatal tests, you will be offered intravenous antibiotics in labour to significantly reduce the chance of your baby contracting GBS. However, GBS is not routinely tested for in most hospitals in the UK. This is because if you are a carrier today, you might not be tomorrow and vice versa, and the risks of antibiotic use may exceed the benefits. The latest guidelines suggest that if you have tested positive in a previous pregnancy, you will be offered intravenous antibiotics in the current pregnancy or a swab near term.

Several large studies are ongoing to see if a bedside test can increase detection or if vaccination against GBS is effective. New microbiology culture techniques are also now recommended which should improve detection rates.

There's lots of information on the Group B Strep website (www.gbss.org.uk), and a patient information leaflet on the RCOG website (www.rcog.org.uk). There are several laboratories offering screenings for around £35 should you want to get yourself tested.

ANTENATAL CLASSES

Antenatal classes can be one of the most exciting parts of your pregnancy. You have a few options available to you: you can either sign up for NHS-run classes, attend classes run by the National Childbirth Trust (NCT), or go private. Either way it is something you'll have to consider early in your pregnancy as in some areas classes can fill up remarkably quickly.

NCT classes

If you fancy joining the NCT and attending its fabled antenatal classes, you need to get your name down quicker than you can say 'natural birth'. The NCT is a membership charity that provides information, support and classes for parents, families and health professionals, and its classes do get booked up very early. There are a variety of courses on offer, including weekends and evenings for couples, and daytime women-only sessions too. Prices start at around £6 an hour – depending on the session and time.

One of the benefits of joining a local NCT class is that you may forge friendships with local mothers who are giving birth around the same time as you, as the classes are organised around due dates. You probably won't get on with all the women there, but then again, do you like every woman you work with in the office? If you find just one like-minded kindred spirit, it'll be worth it for all the support and cappuccinos you can enjoy together once you both have babes in arms.

Another bonus with the NCT is that it has classes at convenient times, so that working parents can attend without having to take time off work. Some people find there is a distinct bias towards natural childbirth and a 'breast is best' attitude towards feeding, although this does depend on the views of your particular teacher. To sign up to NCT classes, go to www.nct.org.uk.

NHS parentcraft classes

The NHS provides 'parentcraft classes', usually in the last 10 weeks of your pregnancy. These take place either at the hospital where you're due to give birth or at a health centre. The number you get varies from hospital to hospital. Recently many hospitals have combined the classes into a smaller number of more detailed sessions, rather than a large number of short classes. The NHS now offers classes in the evenings and at weekends, and involves partners in all or some of the classes. You are allowed to take paid time off to attend antenatal classes, but your partner is not, so you might want to look at what your local hospital offers as soon as you can so that you can book convenient times.

Private classes

If you want, you can also go down the private route. Some companies offer small group sessions and even one-to-one private evening classes in your own home. Check out www.theknowledgeantenatal.com for more information.

Same-sex couple support

Finding and joining a local gay parenting group can be invaluable when you are in a same-sex relationship and expecting a baby together. Even if you don't feel you need it as parents, it will be really valuable for your child to grow up knowing other children with two mums or two dads. You will also have the opportunity to connect with people going through similar issues, and can ask any questions you may have – for example, the pros and cons of both being called 'mummy', or having two separate names.

POSSIBLE COMPLICATIONS

Before you start reading this section, you need to know that we're going to discuss miscarriage, ectopic pregnancy and stillbirths. This isn't to scare you or worry you – it's here so you're fully informed. If you'd rather not read this section, skip ahead to Chapter 2.

Miscarriage

Sadly, one in seven confirmed pregnancies ends in miscarriage, but in reality the figure is much higher – as many as one in four – because many women miscarry even before they know they are pregnant. Early miscarriage is the loss of a baby before 13 weeks, while late miscarriage is considered to be between 13 and 24 weeks. If you lose a baby after 24 weeks it is called a stillbirth (see page 30).

If you have a miscarriage it is likely that you will never know the cause of it. Chromosomal abnormalities in the fetus are believed to cause around 50% of early miscarriages; this is often described as 'nature's way' of dealing with a baby that wouldn't have survived until full term or would have had severe health problems. Other factors that can influence miscarriage include serious structural problems in the baby, physical problems such as a weak cervix, your health and lifestyle, and certain blood clotting disorders. Very occasionally the baby might get an infection in the uterus and die.

Your age has quite a significant influence on your miscarriage risk: women between 25 and 29 have a 12% chance of having a miscarriage, whereas the risk rises to over 50% in women aged 40–44.

If you have already suffered a miscarriage, you are slightly more at risk of experiencing another in a subsequent pregnancy. Ninety-nine percent of miscarriages happen in the first trimester (13 weeks), so the longer your pregnancy progresses, the less likely it is that you will miscarry.

What happens during miscarriage?

You might experience cramping and blood loss like you would during a normal/ heavy period. If you experience bleeding with low abdominal pain, contact your GP or midwife as soon as you can. They will probably arrange for a scan to check whether you have miscarried and, if you have, that there is nothing left in your uterus that could cause infection or further bleeding.

Often you experience no symptoms and only discover your baby has died when you go for a routine scan, when the sonographer may not be able to detect a heartbeat or may discover an empty pregnancy sac with no baby inside. There are now three possible options. The doctor may recommend that you go home and let nature take its course. Or he may recommend you have an operation called surgical management of miscarriage (SMM). This is a surgical procedure carried out under local or general anaesthetic that will remove the pregnancy. It is a simple operation and will usually be performed as a day case. Increasing numbers of units now offer an outpatient suction procedure instead of SMM called MVA – manual vacuum aspiration. This doesn't involve a general anaesthetic or waiting for a bed, so do ask if your hospital offers this. Alternatively, 'medical management' may be offered, whereby you are given tablets, usually two days apart, to make the pregnancy miscarry completely.

Miscarriage is a devastating thing to happen, but remember that most women go on to have successful pregnancies and that there is lots of help and support out there to help you get over your loss, including the charity Tommy's and The Miscarriage Association (see page 261).

It is recommended that you have at least two periods following a miscarriage before you try to get pregnant again. Emotionally, though, you may feel you need to wait longer before trying again.

Threatened miscarriage

Some women will experience bleeding in early pregnancy. If a scan shows that the pregnancy is developing in the uterus their doctor may advise them to 'wait and see'. This is called a threatened miscarriage. While it's absolute torture wondering whether your baby is going to make it or not, it is quite common to experience light bleeding in the first 12 weeks of pregnancy. If it is not accompanied by pain it might well be your body 'settling down' to being pregnant, and in around 50% of cases the baby will be fine. It is important not to rest completely, but you should stop working while you are bleeding and take life slowly.

Is there anything I can do to avoid miscarriage?

If you do experience a miscarriage, don't beat yourself up about it and wonder if it was anything that you did before you knew you were pregnant. There is some evidence to show that smoking, drinking, recreational drug use and excessive caffeine consumption do increase your risk of miscarriage, which is why it's advisable to quit or severely cut down when you are pregnant. Similarly, women who are seriously overweight and those with health problems should get advice before trying to conceive again – it may be that losing weight or improving control of diabetes will improve the chances of a good outcome next time.

Stress has also been shown to play a part, so worrying about what you did or didn't do may put your baby at just as much risk as that daily double shot latte. Just make sure you look after yourself and always follow your doctor's advice.

Ectopic pregnancy

Another possible pregnancy complication is the occurrence of ectopic pregnancies. This is an uncommon occurrence: in England and Wales one pregnancy in 59 is ectopic.

Ectopic means 'in the wrong place', so an ectopic pregnancy is when the pregnancy develops outside the uterus. Ectopic pregnancies can occur in several places – in the ovary, the abdomen, the cervix or the join between the uterus and the Fallopian tube, but most often it occurs in the Fallopian tube. As the pregnancy develops it can cause pain and bleeding, and if it is not recognised quickly enough it can cause the tube to rupture, causing internal bleeding. This can be fatal if it is not treated quickly enough.

Other symptoms of an ectopic pregnancy include pain at the top of the shoulder, pain when you open your bowels or pass urine, diarrhoea, vomiting and dizzy spells. Clearly none of these is specific to ectopics, but if you are pregnant and have not had a scan yet, you should seek medical advice if you experience any of these.

Ectopic pregnancies are usually found between week 4 and week 10. Some ectopic pregnancies are absorbed naturally back into the body, while others can be treated with a drug that causes the cells to stop dividing, meaning the pregnancy shrinks away. However, the majority of ectopic pregnancies will require surgery, where either the pregnancy or the whole Fallopian tube is removed. Sadly, an ectopic pregnancy can never survive.

The emotional stress and potential danger caused by an ectopic pregnancy can be a traumatic experience and will often require a similar grieving process to a miscarriage. For help or advice on ectopic pregnancies, check out www. ectopic.org.uk.

Stillbirth

While most antenatal care is focused on ensuring the pregnancy is progressing normally, around one in 200 babies is stillborn. The term 'stillbirth' means death at, or before, the birth of a baby who is more than 24 weeks. There is not always one single factor that causes a baby to die in the uterus: often it can be a combination of factors, such as congenital abnormalities (that may not always be picked up on a scan) or low birth weight, or sometimes the placenta can start failing towards the end of pregnancy. Some women will already know that their baby is ill or unlikely to survive, as many problems are detected through antenatal tests and scans; other women will stop feeling their baby move or go for a routine scan to be told the devastating news that their baby has died.

There are many excellent organisations that can help you cope with your grief and loss through counselling and advice; start with SANDS (the stillbirth and neonatal death charity), which offers a confidential helpline to provide support – 0808 164 3332.

2

My baby's development: week by week

Imagining your baby growing inside you is one of the most amazing parts of being pregnant. In this chapter we go through a week-by-week account of your baby's progress in your uterus, and what these changes will mean for your body. We'll cover both the physical and emotional aspects of being pregnant.

TRIMESTERS EXPLAINED

'Trimester' is a word you will see and hear regularly during your pregnancy. It is believed that it evolved from the Latin word *trimestris*, meaning 'three months old' ('tri' meaning three and 'mensis' meaning month), and that's what it roughly means in English, too – three months. So your first trimester is weeks 1–12, your second trimester weeks 13–27 and your third trimester weeks 28–40. However, as you'll soon discover, it's weeks rather than trimesters which are regularly used to monitor the progress of your pregnancy. (In some European countries a different dating system is used, so beware not to be confused if you are travelling.)

THE FIRST TRIMESTER

The first trimester is probably the most amazing in terms of your developing baby. The rate at which the cells multiply and change into a growing foetus and support system is nothing short of miraculous, and it's fascinating to know what's happening (particularly as you can't see or feel much at this stage).

Week 1

The date of the first day of your last menstrual period (even though you are not even pregnant yet, this counts as your first week of pregnancy).

Week 2/3

Conception takes place, and after about three or four days of travelling down the fallopian tubes into your uterus the fertilised egg (or zygote) implants deep into the lining to be nourished and begins to grow.

If the sperm carries a Y chromosome, your baby will be a boy. If it's an X chromosome, you'll be having a girl. After implantation, the little bundle of cells will become an embryo. It sits within a fluid-filled cavity that will become the amniotic sac, and the outer cell mass will develop into the placenta.

Week 4 (the week your period doesn't start)

The embryo is now nestling nicely in the uterus lining; the outer cells are branching out like roots to link into your blood supply to nourish the embryo.

Your little embryo is now about the size of a poppy seed. The inner cells now divide into three layers that will form the baby's body. One layer will form your baby's brain, nervous system, skin, ears and eyes. Another layer forms the lungs, stomach and intestine, and the third will form the heart, bones, muscle and blood. A sensitive urine pregnancy test is usually positive at around this time.

It is also quite common at this stage to experience some spotting, or light bleeding, around the time you would normally have your period. It's worth getting any bleeding checked out by your GP.

Week 5: your baby is the size of an apple seed

You may have just found out you are pregnant, but already your baby's nervous system is developing. By the end of this week the top layer of cells have formed a neural tube, which has a 'head end' for the brain and a 'tail end' for the spinal cord. This is why it's advisable to start taking 400 micrograms of folic acid before you conceive, to give you the best chance of preventing neural tube defects such as spina bifida. (Folic acid can be taken as a supplement and is found naturally in leafy vegetables, wholegrain products, berries and fruit.) The embryo resembles a tiny seahorse at this stage.

Your baby is experiencing his first growth spurt. The heart, kidneys and liver are already in place and beginning to form, and blood vessels connecting mother and baby are the beginning of the umbilical cord. Tiny buds that will form his arms and legs are sprouting.

The embryo now becomes safely encased in a bag called the amniotic sac, and is just 4mm–6mm in size.

Mummy matters

Are you feeling sick this week? A recent study suggests that women who suffer badly from morning sickness are more likely to give birth to a baby with a high IQ, as the hormones that cause a woman to vomit are also those that assist in the baby's mental development. There are tips on how to deal with morning sickness on page 68.

Week 6: your baby is the size of a pomegranate seed

This is a period of crucial development for your baby. Your baby's heart is now beating about 150 times a minute, which is twice as fast as yours.

His features are starting to form – his head is very large in proportion to the rest of the developing embryo, and slight depressions can be seen where his eyes, ears and nostrils are growing.

Bulges appear showing the position of the heart, and the heartbeat can be detected on an ultrasound scan.

Week 7: your baby is the size of a blueberry

Your baby's eyes and ears are already starting to form, as are the muscles and bones. His heart and brain are getting more complex, and facial features such as his nose are starting to grow. He doesn't have fingers yet, but his arms are rounded with impressions where the fingers will be.

You may be suffering from fatigue and feeling low on energy, and mood swings are common where you feel joyous one minute and tearful the next. This is a normal result of hormone changes, and will soon pass. However if you experience any cramping or bleeding, you must seek medical help immediately.

Mummy matters

If you are suddenly resembling a spotty teenager with lank greasy hair and zits, don't despair: this phase is usually short lived and is thanks to those hormones running amok in your body. Try to pamper yourself with a warm bath and an at-home facial.

Week 8: your baby is the size of a raspberry

At this point the embryo is now around 1.5cm–2cm long and prawn-shaped. The foot and hand areas can be recognised, as can the fingers and toes, but these may still be webbed. His elbow and knee joints are bending and beginning to curl around his body, and he is taking on a more human shape. The eyes are now becoming visible, the mouth and tongue have formed, and the major organs are developing.

 Mummy matters

Having trouble keeping your eyes open past 9pm? Feeling exhausted is very common in early pregnancy, and is just your body reacting to the effort it takes to set up the life support system for your baby. Listen to your body and rest up as much as you can. Indulge in early nights with a good book, which will be good for your body and your stress levels.

Week 9: your baby is the size of a cherry

All your baby's body parts – arms, legs, organs, eyes – are present by this week, but they are not fully formed. The embryo is now between 2cm–3cm long, measured from head to bottom. This is called the crown–rump length, and is a very accurate way of dating the pregnancy between 7 and 12 weeks. At nine weeks your baby is approximately 2.2cm long, and at 10 weeks, 3.1cm.

Week 10: your baby is the size of a prune

From this stage your baby is referred to as a fetus. He's about 3cm–3.5cm long, and his size will more than double over the next few weeks. All his major organs are now fully developed, and he begins to move his limbs and kick within your uterus, although you can't yet feel anything.

Your baby's head is still disproportionately large, but the body is starting to lengthen. The placenta is now fully formed and transporting nutrients between you and your baby. You will probably be having your first midwife booking appointment around now.

 Mummy matters

During pregnancy your sense of smell is often heightened: certain smells can be quite repulsive, and, equally, strange smells can become quite appealing.

The placenta

The placenta forms from part of the group of cells that implanted into the lining of your uterus shortly after conception. It is the organ that joins you and your baby together via the umbilical cord, and it supplies your baby with all the resources he needs to grow. It allows for the transfer of oxygen, nutrients and antibodies from mother to baby, and for the baby to get rid of waste products. It also means that your baby is born with some immunity against many serious infections that will protect him in the first few weeks of life before he gets his own vaccinations. The circulation of blood for mother and baby are kept completely separate, though. This is a really important part of the placenta's role, particularly if you and your baby have different blood groups, or you need to take certain medications. Problems with the way the placenta works can sometimes cause the baby to be smaller than expected (because the supply of food is less than usual), or can be linked with pre-eclampsia (see page 64).

The placenta grows throughout your pregnancy, and by the time the baby is born it will weigh a whopping half a kilo (just over one pound)! It normally detaches itself after birth and is usually delivered less than 30 minutes after your baby is born via the birth canal. Sometimes the placenta does not deliver spontaneously, and then you might need to have it removed (see page 234) or you may be given an injection to speed up the process.

The placenta is considered to be very important in certain cultures and there are many stories stemming from old traditions surrounding it. Filipinos are said to bury a child's placenta with a book to encourage a bright child. In Cambodia some people wrap the placenta in a banana leaf and place it next to the newborn for three days, before burying it for luck. In some African countries the placenta is swaddled and buried beneath a tree to symbolise ongoing life, and other cultures, such as the Maori, bury the placenta to bind the baby to the ancestral land. In China some people view the placenta as having life-giving properties – even after the baby is born – and it is dried and added to food to enhance energy and activity. Apparently, eating the placenta can also protect you against postnatal depression, but don't feel a failure if you decide not to pursue that piece of advice!

Week 11: your baby is the size of a large lime

This week heralds the end of a critical period of development, and the beginning of a new period of dramatic growth. Your baby's sense of hearing is now developing; his eyes are fully formed but still closed.

His heart is now sufficiently well developed to be pumping his own blood around his body. He has milk (first) teeth buds and toenails, and some of his bones are beginning to harden. He has distinct human characteristics and resembles a baby, which you will be able to see at your scan around now.

He now measures around 4.5cm–6cm.

Week 12: your baby is the size of a large plum

Your baby now weighs about 14g (0.49 oz). Incredibly, your baby is now fully formed, with all the internal organs, muscles, bones and limbs present. The sex organs are also well developed, although they are not visible.

Your baby can now suck, yawn and swallow, but although he is moving around a lot you won't be able to feel it yet.

Your doctor or midwife may be able to feel the top of the uterus in your lower tummy, and that means they may be able to hear your baby's heartbeat. Needless to say, this is a very exciting moment, and tangible evidence that something special is really happening inside you!

 Mummy matters

By this point your breasts will be bigger, so it might be time to invest in a supportive bra. It is advisable that you do not wear an underwire bra during your pregnancy, as your breast tissue is very delicate and expanding fast.

First trimester summary

What has happened so far:

- You have found out the amazing news that you are having a baby.
- You should have visited your doctor or midwife and had a booking appointment with a midwife.
- You may have had a dating and a nuchal scan at around 12 weeks, or a different screening test for Down's syndrome.

Reasons to be cheerful even if you're feeling rough:

- This is a real milestone for pregnant women, because the chances of having a miscarriage after 13 weeks drop to around 1%.
- Your morning sickness symptoms *might* subside – fingers crossed!
- You're creating your own family. Many couples find having a baby brings them even closer together.
- You can feel confident about sharing the news with work colleagues and friends.
- Free dental treatment. Any check-ups and essential work from an NHS dentist won't cost you a penny.
- Free prescriptions.
- Period-free for up to a year – or maybe more!
- You've only got 27 weeks to go.

THE SECOND TRIMESTER

You may have had the incredible experience of 'meeting' your baby via a scan by now, or are certainly just about to. Suddenly the whole pregnancy/having-a-baby concept feels like a reality.

Week 13: your baby is the size of a peach

By this stage your baby will be between 6cm and 8cm in length. Your baby is growing rapidly now and beginning to look more human. He will also have started to develop a fine covering of downy hair called lanugo. Doctors believe the purpose of this hair is to regulate temperature in the uterus; this hair disappears before birth or shortly afterwards. Babies that are born premature are often still covered in this fine, silky hair.

By this stage of pregnancy most women can stop taking folic acid supplements, as the time for formation of the baby's spinal cord and heart is over. It is worth checking with your GP or midwife, though, since some women need to continue a folate supplement throughout the pregnancy.

This a good time to get your GP or midwife to complete form FW8, which should be readily available in the surgery – this confirms that you are pregnant and gets you a Maternity Exemption Certificate (it may be in the form of a paper certificate, a plastic card or an email), which allows you to have free prescriptions and free dental treatment until 12 months after the baby's due date. This only applies to NHS dentists, though, so if you have a private dentist you may still have to pay. If you don't do it now you can get around to it at any point, including after the baby's birth, but to save you money it's worth getting on with it!

Week 14: your baby is the size of a lemon

Your baby is developing his movement, and his muscles are beginning to function. He can now grasp with his fist, frown, squint and grimace. Some day he will be smiling for you!

By now you'll not only have had the first glimpse of your baby, you'll also get the opportunity to hear him too. From around 14 weeks your doctor or midwife can use a Doppler – a handheld monitoring machine – to locate and listen to your baby's heartbeat.

 Words from the professionals

Although you can now buy a Doppler that you can use at home to listen to the baby's heartbeat, the current medical advice is not to be tempted to buy one. Spend your money on something more useful, as it is often difficult to tell the difference between your heartbeat and the baby's – it's also quite difficult to find the heartbeat unless you are trained how to do so.

A normal fetal heart rate (FHR) can be anything between 110 and 160 beats per minute (BPM), but on average it's around 140. This is twice as fast as a normal adult's. The old wives' tale says that a faster heart rate is a girl and a slower heart rate is a boy, but who knows how true that is!

Week 15: your baby is the size of an apple

At this stage your baby weighs around 50g (1.7oz). His fingernails have started growing and his eyes and ears are migrating to the right parts of his head. His legs are lengthening to be more in proportion with his body, and all his joints can move. Meconium (or baby poo) is made in the intestine, but not released yet.

 Words from the professionals

Are your boobs feeling even bigger? From week 15 you might start producing colostrum: the yellow fluid that is meant to nourish your baby during his first few days before the breast milk comes in.

Week 16: your baby is the size of an avocado

From now your baby's hearing is developing, so he can start to hear you talking. His eyes can now perceive light, although the eyelids are still closed. Your baby's limbs are now moving around quite freely, and he might be able to suck his thumb.

 Words from the professionals

Now is a good time to have the whooping cough vaccination, to make sure your baby is born with high enough levels of immunity so that he doesn't catch it while he is very young. Ask your GP for the injection.

Week 17: your baby is the size of a pear

Your baby is now around 13cm long. His eyes are now looking forward. His skeleton is hardening as cartilage changes to bone, and fat is beginning to be laid down. The umbilical cord is getting thicker and stronger. The baby and the placenta are around the same size at this point.

You might begin to feel the first movements, or 'quickening', at this stage. Some say it feels like bubbles or butterflies in your tummy, and it's hard to be sure at this stage whether it's the baby or just wind!

Mummy matters

Good news is that at 17 weeks your hair may start to look thicker and shinier. You may be feeling more energised as your metabolic rate has increased – which might also make you hungrier!

Week 18: your baby is the size of a capsicum pepper

If you were able to shake your baby's hand, you would feel a strong grip. The facial features have now also developed, making him look more human: he can even pull faces! He is yawning and hiccuping, and although you may not be able to feel this yet, you will soon. The hands have developed lines, creating individual fingerprints.

Week 19: your baby is the size of a mango

Lots of soft hair is now appearing on your baby's head, and the eyelashes and eyebrows are growing too.

This is a very important time in your baby's development. Nerve cells, which enable your baby to interact with and comprehend the world, are developing within his brain.

Your pelvic ligaments are softening and abdominal muscles are stretching, so it's never too early to begin practising your pelvic floor exercises (see page 108) to ensure your spine is as supported as possible towards your third trimester.

 Words from the professionals

Now's the time to sign up for a pregnancy yoga or Pilates class, to help maintain abdominal tone and help prevent any pregnancy aches and pains. It also gives you a relaxing hour to focus on yourself and your baby.

Week 20: your baby is the size of a banana

Your baby is now around 18cm long and weighs around 280g (9.8oz).

By now he can hear noises outside the uterus, and shortly will be able to recognise your voice and that of your partner. If you are startled by a loud bang, chances are your baby will jump too. By this stage your baby's gender can be detected on an ultrasound scan.

You might feel your baby's movements now, but some women don't until they are past 20 weeks. If the placenta is located at the front of your uterus (which you will find out at your anomaly scan) it may take longer to feel movements, and it may be difficult to feel them at all as the placenta acts as a sponge at the front between you and your baby. This is not a cause for concern; it just makes it harder to feel movements.

Your baby will now have adopted a sleeping cycle, with peak movements at certain times of the day or night. Once you have established these movements you'll be able to recognise when he is awake or asleep (hopefully at the same time as you!). He sleeps for only 20 to 40 minutes at a time. This sleep pattern is often continued as a newborn, with one sleep cycle lasting 20 minutes.

Around this time you will have an anomaly scan, which checks the structures of your baby and the major organs, as well as the position of the placenta. It also confirms the dates of the pregnancy. See page 19 for more information about this scan.

Week 21: your baby is the size of a pomegranate

Your baby has now started to practise his breathing skills in preparation for birth, by inhaling and exhaling amniotic fluid – this ensures his lungs develop normally.

The taste buds are also developing; it may be an old wives' tale, but apparently your baby can develop a taste for things you eat in your pregnancy (maybe stay off the caviar then …).

His eyebrows and fingernails are fully developed and visible.

At this stage you can collect your MATB1 form from a doctor or midwife. This proves you are pregnant, and is needed by your employer when arranging maternity leave and benefits (see Chapter 5).

 Mummy matters

If you get the odd tummy twinge, don't worry: it's just the ligaments around the womb stretching to accommodate the increase in size. This feels a little like twitching muscles after you have exercised.

Week 22: your baby is the size of a papaya

Your baby's immune system is developing by forming white blood cells to protect against infection.

His head and body size have evened out and his eyes and lips are now more developed, so the fetus is now a small but perfectly formed version of the baby you are going to meet in around 18 weeks' time. His senses are growing as his brain and nerve endings develop, and he may reach up to touch his own face.

The top of your uterus is now around level with your navel and, if you lie down with your head on a pillow and press gently, you may be able to feel it. You will also notice that, as your bump enlarges, your belly button will change shape – this is normal, and caused by the stretching of your skin.

Week 23: your baby is the size of a grapefruit

Your baby now measures around 18cm–20cm.

From this week he begins to put on more and more fat; in a few weeks he will have doubled his weight, and his saggy skin will begin to fill out. He may now be covered with a waxy coating known as vernix, which coats the skin and is believed to protect it from the watery uterus environment (it is your baby's own wetsuit!).

He may get hiccups, which you can now feel! He can also hear and become familiar with all the sounds in your daily life: your favourite music or TV programmes, and the sound of your friends and family. He also has the regular soundtrack of your beating heart, gurgling stomach and whoosh of your blood circulating. This might explain why newborns are soothed by white noise.

Week 24: your baby is the length of an ear of corn

Your baby's see-through skin is still very thin and fragile, but is becoming more opaque. He has eyelashes, although his hair has no pigment yet.

This is a key week, as from 24 weeks it may be possible for a baby to survive if born early, although the chances are slim and unfortunately many of the survivors have significant disabilities. So if you get any symptoms that might be labour – painful cramps in your lower tummy, vaginal bleeding, or leaking of water from the vagina – you should get to your hospital as soon as possible. If you do start to go into labour around this stage of pregnancy, the team looking after you may suggest treatment to try to stop the labour or give you medication to prepare the baby's lungs for breathing and protect his brain. You should have the telephone numbers for your midwife, antenatal clinic and labour ward easily accessible – on the fridge door, stored in your mobile and written in your diary – as you never know when you might need some advice.

Week 25: your baby is the size of a cauliflower

Your baby's lungs should be fully formed around now, and begin to prepare him for his first breath. His tiny nostrils are starting to open so that he can take practice 'breaths' through the nose, in his amniotic environment.

You might think you have a karate black belt in the making, as your baby somersaults, kicks and generally makes his presence felt!

If the area around your nipple (the areola) becomes bigger and darker, this is completely normal and is just your body preparing your breasts for breastfeeding.

Week 26: your baby is the size of an iceberg lettuce

Your baby's brain is now more developed and sophisticated, and he may respond to external stimulus such as sounds and light, and is becoming more active.

He may now be able to open his eyelids for the first time, and his fingernails are growing. His lungs begin to produce surfactant, the substance that allows the air sacs in the lungs to inflate, and stops them collapsing and sticking together when they deflate.

You will usually have a blood test at 26–28 weeks to check for anaemia and possibly diabetes and to confirm your blood group. If your Rhesus blood group is Rhesus negative and your baby's group is predicted to be Rhesus positive or is unknown, you will be given an Anti D injection to ensure you don't have problems with any subsequent pregnancies, should you happen to have a second Rh positive baby – see page 14 for more information.

 Mummy matters

As your baby gets bigger, there will be more pressure on your lower back and legs, so ask a loved one to give you a gentle shoulder massage or foot rub. Alternatively, you can have a long soak in the bath to relieve any aches or pains.

Week 27: your baby is the size of a swede

Your baby is now around 30cm long. His brain is developing rapidly in these weeks, so make sure you are following the best diet you can. It is believed that babies start to dream around this time as they now experience the rapid eye movement (REM) phase of sleep, although it's impossible to know about what!

Your baby can now open and close his eyes, and follow more regular patterns of sleep and wakeful time. He is now 'breathing' with fully functioning lungs. In the unlikely event of your going into premature labour, if he was born from this week there is a greater chance of his survival.

Second trimester summary

What has happened so far:

- You will have had a second, more detailed, anomaly scan to check everything is progressing well.
- You can now know the gender of your baby if you want to.

Reasons to be cheerful even if you're feeling rough:

- You should now have quite a pronounced bump, and hopefully strangers are giving up their seats for you on public transport.
- Shopping: it's a good time to start buying essentials for your baby, in case you do slow down a bit towards the end of the pregnancy.
- Your baby has a reasonable chance of survival if born after 28 weeks.
- If you want to, you can go on maternity leave in just a couple of weeks.

 Mummy matters

By this stage things are getting real. Your baby will be earthside in a matter of weeks, so don't be worried if your emotions range from, 'I'm so excited I think I'm going to explode!' to, 'Oh my word, what have I done?' You are bound to be anxious about the birth and how you are going to cope, and these feelings are both natural and understandable.

Planning your baby's upbringing

Thinking about the way you will bring your child up might also be occupying your thoughts at this stage in the pregnancy; it's a good time to talk over issues with your partner, because you might find that once you have had the baby you haven't got the time or energy to discuss such matters. For example, different religious beliefs can cause conflict when it comes to raising a child, so it's good to iron out any potential disagreements before they become insurmountable problems within your relationship.

You and your partner might want to talk about your own childhoods, and figure out the things that made you happiest, as undoubtedly you will want the same things for your child. There might also be things in your own upbringing – like never sitting down to dinner as a family – that you look back on with regret, and you might vow not to make the same mistakes as your parents (though once you become one you will quickly learn that *nobody* is perfect).

Considering how your relationship will change

The end of the second trimester is a brilliant time to really look at how a baby is going to change your life, and how you are going to have to adapt to accommodate this new person in your relationship.

Talk about the aspects of your life that you think will change. The more you have prepared yourself for the kinds of adjustments and sacrifices you may have to make, the less of a shock it will be. Plan to make time for each other as a couple and to be honest about your feelings.

THE THIRD TRIMESTER

You've reached the last trimester, where you'll be preparing for your baby's arrival, and coping with your ever-growing bump.

Week 28: your baby is the size of a large aubergine

Your baby's eyes are now moving around in their sockets, and if you were to shine a bright light on your bump he would probably turn to look at it.

About half of all babies have by now moved into an optimum position for birth: head down. There is still plenty of time for him to move if he hasn't, though. Your baby is interacting more with you, so now's the time to start singing him lullabies or reading stories.

Your baby should weigh just over 1kg (2lb), so he now weighs the same as a bag of sugar! He's developing more fat as weeks go on, so his skin is less wrinkly now.

You might start feeling Braxton Hicks contractions (an irregular tightening of the uterus lasting around 30 to 60 seconds) at this stage. Normally they last no more than 30 seconds and don't become stronger or more frequent, like proper contractions. They are nothing to worry about unless they become more painful or occur often or at regular intervals, or if there is any vaginal bleeding or leaking of fluid, in which case you might be at risk of pre-term labour and should seek medical advice. If you're at all concerned, contact your doctor or midwife.

Week 29: your baby is the size of a butternut squash

Your baby's translucent skin is beginning to turn opaque, and pinker due to capillaries under the skin. His bones are fully formed, although still very soft.

He is moving around but there is now less room in the uterus, so rather than vigorous kicks and somersaults you might begin to feel more of a poke in the ribs from his elbow or knee.

Week 30: your baby is the length of a cucumber

By now your baby is about 33cm long and gaining weight, making him look smoother and less wrinkly. The hair on his head should be growing. His brain is growing and developing. He is now able to form a strong fist and grasp. From around now he starts to shed his lanugo, the downy hair that covers his body, as he is more able to regulate his own body temperature.

 Mummy matters

If you are at risk of varicose veins (if your mum got them in pregnancy it's likely you will too), it might be worth investing in a pair of support tights – particularly if you are on your feet all day. You may feel like Nora Batty but it might keep the varicosities and mild ankle swelling in check.

Week 31: your baby is the size of a coconut

Your baby's lungs are fully formed and are capable of breathing air, but need more time to mature. If he is a boy, his testicles are moving through the groin towards the scrotum.

He's nearly at his birth length; now it's all about putting on more baby fat under the skin. His brain is more sophisticated: processing information, following light, and interpreting through all five senses.

Now is a good time to start making a birth plan if you haven't already done so. This can include anything that is important to you during the labour and delivery. There is probably a section in your hospital notes giving you an idea of the types of questions you should be asking yourself: 'Who do I want to be with me?', 'What type of pain relief might I want?', 'What positions do I think might be comfortable for me during labour?', 'Am I happy to have a student midwife or medical student involved during my delivery?'. Make some notes about what you think might be good for you and discuss them with your midwife – she will talk through with you what will work and what might not. We look at birth plans in more detail on page 157.

Week 32: your baby is the size of a turnip

There's less space in your uterus and less amniotic fluid, so your baby's pushes and shoves may begin to feel more uncomfortable for you. His immune system is developing and he is receiving your antibodies through the placenta, to enable him to fight off germs in his first crucial few weeks after birth.

Around now, you may be having trouble sleeping. Having a big tummy can make it quite difficult to get comfortable at night, so try propping a couple of pillows under your bump or between your knees as you lie on your side. You could also treat yourself to one of those V-shaped pillows: they're great for breastfeeding and can help support babies when they first sit up, so many women think they're worth every penny! It's better not to sleep on your back – the weight of your bump can squash the main blood vessel (the vena cava) taking blood back to your heart, and this in turn can reduce the supply of oxygen to you or even your baby. If you do wake up and find you are on your back, don't panic, but do ease a pillow or bit of duvet under your hips and back so that you roll slightly to your left. Also, always try to make sure you get out of bed slowly and carefully – you may feel that your days of jumping out of bed in a lively fashion are over for a while, but even if they are not, you should aim to get up in stages, so that you don't get too dizzy.

 Words from the professionals

Sleeping on your side in the last few months of pregnancy reduces the chance of late stillbirth. The miscarriage, stillbirth and premature birth charity Tommy's have produced a useful video, which can be found at: www.tommys.org/pregnancy-information/sleep-side/sleep-side-late-pregnancy-campaign-film.

Week 33: your baby is the size of a pineapple

Your baby is more likely to have turned around and be facing downwards in preparation for birth. He's keeping his eyes open while he's awake, and is starting to co-ordinate breathing with sucking and swallowing.

Week 34: your baby is the size of a cantaloupe melon

The development of the brain and nervous system is now much more advanced, and most babies born at this stage will survive and be healthy. The baby's head has two soft areas called fontanelles, which allow the skull bones to overlap each other as the baby's head changes shape during its journey through the birth canal. These fontanelles close by the time your baby is two years old. In labour, they are used by the midwife or doctor examining you to work out which way the baby's head is facing.

Your baby is urinating about a pint a day! It is at this stage that baby boys' testicles become visible as they descend into the scrotum.

 Mummy matters

Started tidying obsessively? This nesting instinct is incredibly strong, and we've yet to meet a pregnant woman who didn't admit to having the urge to put her whole house in order.

Feeling your baby move

Those amazing initial flutters that you felt a few months ago have grown into full-blown kicks. It is usual for the frequency of movements to increase until around week 33, and then they plateau for the rest of the pregnancy. If you think your baby's movements have **reduced**, the latest advice from the Royal College of Obstetricians and Gynaecologists is to contact your maternity unit straight away. Usually there is no particular reason why the movements are less frequent, but you should always check it out straight away, since occasionally it is your baby's way of indicating that he is not as well as he should be. Usually it's because he has rolled into a position where the limbs are facing towards you rather than away from you, or perhaps you have had a busy or stressful day and not noticed them as much as usual.

Most maternity departments will have a Day Assessment Unit, which does as the name suggests – usually a friendly and relaxed place, where you can see a midwife (and if required, a doctor) without a formal appointment for a non-emergency query – so it's not the place to go if you think you are in labour or you are bleeding. But if you need an extra blood pressure check, some advice about your backache, or if the baby's movements are not as frequent as usual, it's ideal. You should put the telephone number on the list of useful numbers on the fridge and in your mobile.

 Mummy matters

During pregnancy, it takes a while longer for the blood to overcome gravity and get up to your brain when you stand up. This can include when you have been sitting down on the bus, in the cinema, at a meeting, or when you're getting out of bed: so take it easy.

Week 35: your baby is the size of a honeydew melon

Your baby is building up fat deposits under the skin, which help him keep warm after he is born. He can gain up to half a pound a week at this stage.

If you were to go into labour now, the good news is that the majority of babies born at this stage will be perfectly healthy.

His hearing is fully developed by now, so you might like to sing nursery rhymes or play your favourite songs to your bump. He responds best to high-pitched sounds.

Week 36: your baby is the size of a romaine lettuce

Your baby will now be about 48cm long and weigh nearly 2.8kg (6lb). His kidneys are fully developed. His toenails and fingernails are fully grown. His skin is smoother and his gums are harder. His circulatory and musculoskeletal systems, like most others, are in working order now, although his digestive system won't be fully functioning until he is born and takes in his first milk.

Your baby might 'engage' this week. This is when the head drops down into the pelvis in readiness for birth. It happens earlier in first babies than subsequent ones, and later in women of African descent than women of other races, due to the typical shape of their pelvis.

If your placenta was lying low at the anomaly scan, you will probably be offered another scan around this stage to see if it has changed position. In fact, the placenta itself does not actually move. In the second half of the pregnancy, the lower section of the uterus begins to grow: this means that if the placenta is attached to the upper part of the uterus (which it frequently is), it can be carried higher and away from the cervix. If it is still low, then your doctor will talk though your options with you. If the placenta is blocking the way out for the baby, then you usually need to deliver by Caesarean section. But occasionally, even at this late stage, there may be enough growth in the uterus to allow the baby's head into the pelvis.

Week 37: your baby is the size of a stalk of swiss chard

You are now officially at term. Your baby is likely to be born any time from 37 weeks onwards.

He is practising for entering the world, inhaling and exhaling amniotic fluid, blinking and sucking his thumb in preparation for suckling at the breast or bottle. Everything he swallows is creating meconium, his first dark sticky poo, ready for when he is born.

You should have packed your bag (see page 212 for further information on what to pack) so that you are ready for when you go into labour.

Don't worry too much about religiously watching the calendar for your due date. Some say it would be better not to give a 'due date', but rather a 'due period' – it raises too many expectations, and, as you are probably about to find out, is only occasionally the day on which the baby actually arrives! Expect your baby to arrive between 37 and 42 weeks: that is, three weeks before and two weeks after the so-called due date.

 Mummy matters

Cover your mattress with a towel or protector just in case your waters break during the night.

Your baby will probably have lost all the lanugo and vernix by now.

Your midwife, GP or obstetrician will be keeping a close eye on the position of your baby, as he should be head down from 37 weeks and ready for when labour starts – which could be any day now. But 5% of babies are not head down by this stage, so be prepared for some poking! If the baby is lying bottom or feet first (breech) there are various methods doctors and midwives can use to try to make him turn (see page 208). If the baby can't be turned, or decides to flip back, then the team looking after you should discuss the pros and cons of a breech vaginal birth or a Caesarean section with you, and help you make the safest choice for you and the baby. Some babies are breech until the day before labour starts and decide to turn at the last minute, so don't worry too much if your baby isn't where he should be at the moment.

If your baby is lying sideways, or 'transverse', after 37 weeks, your doctor will want to find out why (for example, something else in your pelvis may be taking the space meant for the baby's head – such as the placenta), and may suggest you stay in hospital. One of the important things about your baby's head or bottom being in the pelvis at the time that labour starts is that, if the waters break, it can act as a 'plug' and stop the umbilical cord washing down into the vagina and out of your body before the baby does.

One of the benefits of your baby moving down into your pelvis is that you might be able to breathe more easily, as there is more lung capacity now he has moved down a little! Also, your heartburn might not be quite so bad. On the other hand, there will be even more pressure on your bladder and pelvis, so getting a good night's sleep won't be any easier as you will need to go to the toilet more often. Some say that is all good preparation for the sleepless nights of new parenthood!

Week 38: your baby is the size of a pumpkin

Your baby should weigh around 3kg (7lb) now. He's still building up his layer of fat, which will help him to regulate his own temperature when he enters the outside world.

Week 39: your baby is the size of a watermelon

Your baby is now able to fully flex his limbs now. His nails may be slightly overgrown and need a trim by the time he comes out! If you need a planned Caesarean section, this is the most common time for one to be booked – it is a balance of minimising the chance of you going into labour and maximising the baby's chance of staying out of the Special Care Baby Unit (SCBU).

Week 40

Hopefully, the waiting is nearly over and you'll give birth pretty soon, although less than 5% of babies arrive on their due date and only 30% in the week around your due date, so don't fret if he doesn't make an appearance just yet.

 Words from the professionals

Many pregnancies go on to 40 weeks and beyond. If you are still pregnant, put your feet up, try to relax and make the most of those extra days of peace and quiet: you're going to need them! If you are over 40 years old or conceived by IVF, your team might suggest induction nearer 40 weeks than 42.

Week 41

At this stage your midwife might suggest doing a 'sweep'. This isn't part of the nesting activity we discussed earlier; it's a way of encouraging labour to start naturally. It involves having an internal examination, which allows the midwife to stretch the cervix (the neck of the uterus) and sweep the membranes of the amniotic sac away from the cervix, thereby releasing the natural chemicals called prostaglandins which are involved in the initiation of labour. It can be a bit eye-watering, but it will be worth it if labour starts spontaneously.

If the sweep doesn't do the trick, then towards the end of week 41 you will usually be offered induction of labour. There is evidence to suggest that women who labour after 42 weeks are less likely to have a vaginal delivery than those who labour earlier. There is also evidence that the placenta is less likely to function normally after 42 weeks, and this slightly increases the (small) chance of stillbirth. Most units will have an information sheet about induction for you to read, and will be happy to talk it through in as much detail as you need. Some women are so exhausted by the pregnancy at this stage that they welcome the opportunity to finally get things going, while others are reluctant to disturb a natural process.

If you are told you may need to be induced, make sure you get all the information you need and feel comfortable with what the procedure will involve. See page 223 for more information about induction.

Third trimester summary

You've done it! You've got through the past 40 weeks and it might have been a struggle at times but boy, it will have been worth it … we promise.

3

My body: pains and pampering

Growing a baby inside of you is nothing short of a miracle – however, you'll more likely than not experience some uncomfortable and often embarrassing side effects that you might not have been expecting. Here we look at the most common problems and how you can make yourself a bit more comfortable.

It's worth bearing in mind while you're reading through all the various afflictions that can strike during pregnancy that, for every 'bad' element of pregnancy, there's a 'good' one too – glossy hair, fabulous bosoms, beautiful belly – so we also look at the fantastic 'side effects' of being pregnant: how your body changes shape and the other bonus features of having a bun in the oven!

We know that certain factors, such as age and general health, will affect how your body reacts to pregnancy, but a great deal is down to genetics, hormones and good (or bad) luck!

ACHES AND PAINS

The good news is that most of the pain you experience in pregnancy is completely normal and harmless; indeed, it would be quite surprising if you didn't experience pangs or twinges, given the weight and complexity of the cargo you are carrying. Below, we take a look at the different areas of your body that may be affected and suggest ways to make you feel more comfortable.

Words from the professionals

On page 80 is a list of symptoms that might need urgent advice or attention. If you are very worried and you can't get through to a midwife – your hospital emergency number should be on your notes – call NHS 111, get to the labour ward or A&E (if you are less than 18 weeks) if someone can take you, or dial 999 for an ambulance.

Abdominal pain

It is not unusual to experience some abdominal pain in pregnancy and, although it might worry you, generally there is no cause for alarm. Wind and constipation are common and so is a loosening of the pelvic bone where it joins at the front. Some women find that they experience a period-like pain at the beginning of pregnancy as the embryo implants in the uterus. This is often a constant dull ache and feels a little like a muscle strain.

From the second trimester onwards, you might feel a sharp twinge in your side or groin area as the muscles and ligaments around your uterus stretch.

In the third trimester it can be normal to experience Braxton Hicks or 'practice' contractions as your body prepares itself for labour. Remember that you are probably much more in tune with your body now than you were before you were pregnant, and so what you are feeling may be normal, but you just didn't notice or respond to it before!

What can I do?
If you are experiencing pains in your tummy, the best advice is to sit and rest until they subside.

 Words from the professionals

If you have a severe or persistent abdominal pain you should get yourself checked out immediately, especially if you experience vaginal bleeding. If it happens in the first 12 weeks, it could be a sign of miscarriage or an ectopic pregnancy (see pages 27–30); up to 24 weeks, it could be a late miscarriage; and from then on, it could indicate you are going into early labour. It's also possible that the pain might be due to another cause unrelated to pregnancy – like appendicitis – that needs urgent medical attention. The most common cause unrelated to pregnancy is a urine infection. You should contact your GP, midwife or labour ward straightaway if you experience persistent pain, especially if it is associated with bleeding.

Back pain

Back pain will affect as many as 75% of pregnant women at some point during their pregnancy. It tends to get worse in the third trimester, as the body releases a hormone called relaxin to make the joints and ligaments in the pelvic region more flexible in preparation for birth. The downside of this hormone is that it makes the body more susceptible to pain and injury. As you are carrying a lot of extra weight at the front your posture is affected, meaning your back curves more (to stop you toppling forward!) and tends to take the strain. Protecting your back is another reason not to gain too much weight while you are pregnant and a really important reason to lose it again after delivery.

The good news is that, for most women, back problems do ease after birth, although labour itself can sometimes be a strain on your back – make sure your midwife helps you to look after it in labour. Relaxin can stay in your system for some time, so you should protect your back by learning the best way to pick up your newborn. Always bend at your knees and hips, keeping your back straight, and don't twist.

What can I do?

- Gentle exercise like swimming, yoga and Pilates can strengthen muscles and prevent or ease backache.
- If you sit at a desk all day, make sure that your computer and chair are at the correct height (it may need to change as your bump expands).
- Pay attention to your posture and try not to stand for long periods. You should also ditch your heels and switch to flats.
- Avoid lifting anything heavy, and if you do need to pick up anything weighty make sure you bend your knees.
- Try a maternity band or belt – a stretchy fabric band that sits underneath the bump and supports it.

Words from the professionals

Paracetamol can be used safely in pregnancy if your back pain warrants it, but avoid ibuprofen, Nurofen and other painkillers from the same group (which are called nonsteroidal anti-inflammatory drugs), unless you have discussed it directly with your doctor.

Physiotherapy can be helpful: ask your doctor whether a referral might help you.

If you get any signs of sciatica (that is, compression of one of the nerves to the legs as it leaves the spinal column), such as shooting pains in the legs or buttocks (most commonly on one side only and not on both), weakness, or numbness in part of the leg, discuss this with your doctor.

Pelvic/pubic pain

When you give birth your pelvis, which is normally stable, widens slightly to make more room for the baby. Sometimes a combination of the weight of the baby and the loosening of the pelvic ligaments means that this widening, or separation, of the pelvic bones occurs prior to delivery, and sometimes this is painful – referred to as symphysis pubis dysfunction (SPD) or pelvic girdle pain (PGP). Usually the pain is in the lowest part of your tummy, in the midline: if you gently press with two fingers in that area, through the triangle of pubic hair, you should feel the bone. This is where the two sides of the pelvis join together (called the pubic symphysis), and it is unusual movement in the joint that causes pain. If you press too hard, it may feel tender. When your midwife or doctor examines you, they may measure the size of your bump, and the discomfort that you feel when they press at the bottom of your tummy is due to softening in the pubic symphysis. This can occur at any time in the second half of your pregnancy, and the pain may vary from mild to very troublesome. It is likely to be particularly uncomfortable when you open your legs wide apart, such as when getting out of bed or out of the car; you may also find sex a bit tricky! It can involve your buttocks, thighs or hips, and some women report that they feel a clicking sensation when they walk.

When it is severe it can make everyday activities, such as walking, driving and climbing stairs, torturous. This does not usually affect how you give birth, but talk to your midwife if you are concerned. The good news is that the pelvic bones normally go back into their proper position after birth and the pain improves.

What can I do?

Keep your knees together *all* the time and keep gently mobile if you can, even if it is at a slow and cautious pace. You may have to stop work earlier than you had planned. A pelvic support belt can also help to relieve the pressure on the pelvis.

 Words from the professionals

Obstetric physiotherapists will teach you exercises to ease the symptoms of SPD, and, even more importantly, positions to adopt and avoid. They may give you a 'girdle', rather like a massive tubigrip over your pelvis, which can help stabilise the joint. Sometimes safe painkillers such as paracetamol are helpful. If things get really bad, your doctor will offer advice on how to manage the discomfort. A few women need crutches.

Sometimes, SPD can drive women to beg for induction of labour. If it gets that bad for you, do talk with your doctor or midwife. However, usually it is not necessary to do this, and certainly the extra vaginal examinations that are required for induction can be very difficult for you.

If you have SPD, your midwife will look after your pelvis and support your hips appropriately in labour. You may need to review your thoughts about pain relief, since the combination of SPD pain and labour can sometimes be quite wearing. Epidurals and SPD can go very well together!

Cramp

It is common to experience leg cramps during pregnancy. They can be intensely painful, and occur when a muscle or group of muscles go into spasm – you will find that the offending muscles have gone rock hard, and might pull your leg or foot into an odd shape.

There isn't a clear medical explanation for their occurrence, although theories include muscle fatigue, dehydration, mineral deficiency, and pressure on the nerves caused by the growing uterus.

What can I do?

- If you do get an attack of cramp, stretch out your leg or foot to counteract the way the muscle is pulling. For example, if you have cramp in the bottom of your foot (a really common site) you will probably need to pull your foot up towards your body – as your bump gets bigger, this is not as easy as it sounds, so you may need to engage the help of a supportive partner or best friend.

- Sometimes you can walk off cramps, like you might with pins and needles.

- Avoid sitting with your legs crossed.

- Give your muscles a firm rub if they go into spasm, or ask someone to do it for you.

(🧬) Words from the professionals

If the cramps are really bothering you, it might be worth chatting to your doctor or midwife, because you might be missing some minerals in your diet – but don't take a supplement without their advice.

If you have persistent pain, or other symptoms such as leg swelling or reddening of the painful leg, contact your GP as it could be a sign of something more serious like deep vein thrombosis (see page 65).

Hand pain

Carpal tunnel syndrome is caused by a build-up of fluid in the wrist, which means that the nerve passing through to the hand is compressed. It can affect as many as one in three pregnant women. Symptoms include numbness, pins and needles, stiffness, and varying degrees of pain in your hands and fingers (and especially the thumb, index and middle fingers), which is often worse in the mornings. When you have been lying down overnight your ankles will usually become less swollen. This is because the fluid that collected in them under the influence of gravity by day has redistributed by night, and some is now in your wrists (although usually you cannot see the swelling in the wrists, unlike the situation in your ankles!).

In general it begins to get better after delivery, but may take quite a few weeks – if there is no improvement by the time your baby is ready for his six-week check-up, ask your doctor about it at the same time.

What can I do?

- Curl your fingers into a fist and then straighten them out several times; bend your hand to and fro at the wrist repeatedly to try to ease away the fluid.

- Bend your hands at the wrist so that the backs of your fingers extend up towards your forearm.

- Stretch out and relax your fingers several times.

- Raise your hands whenever you can and try to sleep with them on the pillow.

- Don't handle the family heirlooms – you may have turned into a butterfingers!

 Words from the professionals

Your doctor may refer you to physiotherapy. They may give you a support brace to wear on your wrist at night, holding it in the extended position described above – it is quite hard to sleep with these on, though, so you may choose just to put up with it!

Headaches

There are a myriad of reasons why you might suffer from headaches in pregnancy: hormones and changes in blood supply are considered to be the most likely culprits, but other factors such as dehydration, nausea, insomnia, nasal congestion and stress may also play a part.

What can I do?

- If you have a headache or feel one coming on, try taking a rest in a darkened room.

- You are probably aware you should avoid painkillers such as ibuprofen while you are pregnant. Current advice remains that it is safe to take paracetamol.

- If you are prone to headaches, take preventative measures by keeping yourself hydrated, following a good diet and getting as much rest and sleep as you can.

- It's a good idea to cut your caffeine consumption, or try some decaf tea or coffee, particularly if you get headaches regularly. (It is recommended that you drink no more than two cups of caffeinated drinks a day when pregnant.)

 Words from the professionals

Headaches are not normally serious, but if you experience severe or frequent head pains/migraines or if they are accompanied by blurred vision, vomiting or swelling, you should see your midwife or GP straightaway as it could be a sign of pre-eclampsia (see page 64).

Rib pain

It is quite normal to experience some rib pain, especially in the third trimester. You may feel it at the sides or where the ribs join the breast bone at the front. The ribs move upwards in pregnancy: partly pushed by the expanding uterus, and partly because of the deeper breaths that you automatically make in order to take in extra oxygen for the baby. You might also feel some discomfort when your baby gives you a swift left hook in the rib cage as space gets really tight. The good news is that once your baby's head engages, pressure on the rib area subsides.

What can I do?

Try to maintain good posture and support yourself with cushions when sitting for long periods of time.

BLOOD CHANGES

Some pregnancy symptoms are caused by changes in the blood as it works overtime to support both you and your growing baby. Here are some of the most common problems you might encounter and some tips on how to relieve your discomfort.

Anaemia

Anaemia is a lack of haemoglobin in the red blood cells in the body. Haemoglobin carries oxygen around the body, and in the placenta it passes oxygen across to the fetus. Pregnant women increase their production of both haemoglobin and red blood cells during pregnancy, in order to carry the extra oxygen needed by the developing fetus and to provide the mother with the oxygen needed for the growth and development of her body. To produce these new red blood cells, the body needs extra iron, vitamin B12 and folic acid, and if there is a deficiency in any of these ingredients anaemia can develop. Pregnant women also pass iron to the placental tissue and to the fetus, which can lead to anaemia.

Often anaemia has no symptoms: this is one reason why you will be asked for a blood sample both at your booking appointment and around week 28 of pregnancy. The signs of anaemia include tiredness and paleness; you might also experience exhaustion, dizziness and palpitations, although all of these are common in pregnancy anyway.

It is really important to prevent and/or treat anaemia in pregnancy. There is some evidence that babies of mothers who lacked iron during pregnancy have less well-developed brains. Blood loss at delivery is also relatively common, and if you are anaemic before you go into labour, you are much more likely to need a blood transfusion after delivery.

What can I do?
To help you avoid or alleviate anaemia, try to eat:

- foods that are particularly rich in iron (such as wholemeal bread, cereals, spinach, eggs, dried fruits and lean meat)

- a diet rich in vitamin C (oranges, lemons and raw vegetables) as it helps your body absorb iron. Try to avoid tea and chapattis with your iron-rich foods, since they prevent absorption of the iron from your gut.

- beans, broccoli, asparagus, peas and brussels sprouts, as these are all a good source of folic acid

- meat, dairy products and yeast extract (such as Marmite), as these are good sources of vitamin B12.

 Words from the professionals

If you think you might be anaemic, your doctor or midwife will confirm the diagnosis with a blood test and may prescribe iron tablets. Unfortunately they can cause constipation or diarrhoea, so you might need to try a couple of brands until you find one that works for you. You can also buy natural forms of iron supplements such as Spatone and Floridix. It is commonly said that they don't cause these side effects, but that is only because they don't contain much iron! You need to take very large volumes to get enough iron. If you are taking iron supplements you should take them with fresh orange juice, as vitamin C helps the body to absorb the iron. You also shouldn't have caffeine or milk within an hour of taking them as calcium and caffeine stop the absorption of iron. If your anaemia is severe, your doctor may suggest that iron is given directly into your blood, as an infusion.

Severe anaemia can increase the likelihood of you needing a blood transfusion if you suffer heavy bleeding after birth, so expect your doctor or midwife to keep an eye on your iron levels if you do become anaemic. Severe anaemia can also cause developmental problems for your baby. If you have a fundamental religious belief against blood transfusion (eg Jehovah's Witness) discuss this with your doctor as early as possible in pregnancy.

Fainting

The pressure of the uterus on blood vessels which take blood from the legs back to the heart and lungs means that standing up quickly after sitting or lying can make you dizzy. The blood is still in your legs and takes a while to overcome gravity and get up to your brain, which is why lying down again, on your side, can help. It is also a good idea, when you can, to rest on your left side or in a partially supported position, rather than lying flat on your back, because then the weight of your baby is not compressing your blood vessels as much.

When you are hot, dehydrated or standing still for too long, you can also get dizzy – the blood vessels in the legs accommodate too much blood and there is not enough left to be pumped up to your brain. Again, lying down can help, as can flight stockings. Try to walk on the spot if you have to stand in a queue or on a bus, as the muscles in your calves help to keep the blood flowing around properly.

Although fainting can be quite frightening if it happens when you are out and about, it's not unusual to have a wobbly moment or even a full-on swoon during pregnancy.

What can I do?

- Make sure you stay well hydrated.

- Dress yourself in layers that you can peel off when you find yourself getting too warm.

- In the later stages of pregnancy, ask to leave work earlier so you're not battling public transport when you are tired and hungry.

- If you get that hot flush at the back of your neck and feel yourself about to 'go', sit or lie down immediately. If you are at home, you should lie with your legs raised or sit with your head between your knees (only suitable in early pregnancy as your bump will get in the way later).

Words from the professionals

If you are fainting or feeling dizzy regularly it could be a sign of anaemia, so mention it to your midwife or doctor. Sometimes wearing flight stockings to compress the lower legs is helpful as it stops blood collecting there.

Hot flushes

The increased blood flow around the body and greater metabolic activity of pregnancy produce a lot of extra heat that needs to be dispersed. This can be quite comforting in the chilly winter months; suddenly you've got warm toes in bed. But it can be downright miserable if you are heavily pregnant in the middle of a summer heat wave. Some pregnant women feel warm all over, whereas others suffer classic hot flushes where the face in particular becomes a rather fetching shade of puce.

Another rather unwelcome side effect of overheating is that you may find yourself sweating a lot. Perspiration is the body's way of getting rid of excess heat, so you might want to slap on the deodorant more vigorously than usual.

What can I do?

- Wear natural fibres as they keep the body cool.
- Wear loose clothing.
- Layer up so you can add or remove clothing easily.
- Keep windows open so you can have some fresh air – much healthier than air conditioning – and if you are cooped up in an office all day make sure you pop out at lunchtime (though sit in the shade if it's summertime).
- Drink lots of fluid – ideally water – as your thirst levels rise with your body temperature.

 Words from the professionals

It is known that a severe rise in body temperature can be harmful to your baby, which is why you are advised to get your temperature down quickly if you have a fever. You are advised not to take saunas when pregnant, but this is as much because of the dizziness that can come on in hot places as because of the heat itself. However, there doesn't seem to be anything to suggest that 'normal' pregnancy warmness or heat waves have a detrimental effect on your baby. If you're at all worried, though, speak to your midwife or doctor.

Itching

Itching can be normal in pregnancy and may affect one in four women. It is caused by increased blood flow to, and the stretching and dryness of, your skin, especially over your belly. In late pregnancy your tummy can become itchy because the skin is so stretched over your bump, and sometimes hormones can make your stretch marks more sensitive and more prone to rashes and itchy patches.

What can I do?

- If your skin is itchy, wear loose soft clothing such as a cotton jersey, and use pure cotton bedding.

- If you do have patches of inflamed skin, use something gentle and soothing, such as calamine lotion.

- If you have dry skin, use a water barrier cream such as Diprobase before you bathe or swim to protect your skin from the damaging effects of water.

- Avoid perfumed skin and bath products; stick to simple soaps.

🐣 Words from the professionals

Persistent or severe itching, particularly on the palms of the hands and soles of the feet, can indicate a potentially serious liver condition called obstetric cholestasis or intrahepatic choleostasis, where the liver temporarily works less well. Other symptoms may include dark urine, pale stools, appetite loss and tiredness. If you experience itching, particularly in the third trimester, contact your doctor or midwife. You will usually need a bile acid blood test to try to determine if you have obstetric cholestasis or just itchy dry skin. As severe intrahepatic cholestasis with peak bile acid concentrations over 100 is associated with a small increase in the rate of stillbirth, you may be offered an earlier induction. Latest research suggests that women with mildly elevated bile acids up to 100 do not need early induction. See www.rcog.org.uk for a useful patient information leaflet on obstetric cholestasis.

Nasal congestion and nosebleeds

The increased blood supply driven by those raging hormones puts pressure on the blood vessels inside your nose and causes the sinuses to produce more mucus. This makes your nose more prone to bleeding, congestion and (unfortunately) snoring too.

What can I do?

- If you get a nosebleed, sit upright and pinch the top of your nose gently but firmly for up to 10 minutes. This should stem the bleeding; if not, repeat the process.

- Blow your nose gently to avoid nosebleeds.

- Steam inhalation can help with congestion. Carefully fill a bowl with boiling water, point your face down towards the water, place a towel over your head and the rim of the bowl so you effectively seal in all the steam, and take a few deep breaths. Be warned, though, this technique can make an already flushed face even hotter!

 Words from the professionals

Nosebleeds are generally harmless, but if they are frequent or very heavy you might be at risk of developing anaemia, so do mention them to your doctor if you are suffering badly.

Bleeding in pregnancy

In the first three months you may experience:

- implantation bleeding. Also called 'spotting', this happens a couple of days after conception as the embryo implants itself in the uterus.

- breakthrough bleeding. Light bleeding or spotting when your period would have been due (and occasionally subsequent periods).

- bleeding can also, sadly, be a signal of a serious pregnancy problem such as miscarriage, ectopic or molar pregnancy (see pages 27–30). You should seek medical advice.

After the first three months bleeding is much less common, and tends to have a different list of possible causes, so if you start bleeding you should always inform your midwife and/or doctor as soon as possible. Important causes of bleeding in the second half of pregnancy include:

- placenta praevia. When the placenta is positioned low down in the uterus over the cervix, it is more likely to cause severe bleeding, which is typically painless.

- placental abruption. A rare complication where the placenta separates from the implantation site. Can be life threatening to mother or baby and often necessitates delivery by an emergency Caesarean section. Typically very painful.

- a bloody 'show' could indicate that labour is imminent. After 37 weeks this would be considered normal; before 37 weeks you might be heading for a premature delivery, so you should get to hospital as soon as you can.

There is also a long list of fairly harmless causes of vaginal bleeding, including the following.

- Cervical ectropion (previously called an erosion). This doesn't mean it is damaged or eroded, but that changes in pregnancy make the cervix more prone to harmless bleeding. If you experience light bleeds after sex this could be the cause.

- Vaginal infections, such as thrush, can cause bleeding as well as discharge.

- Benign growths such as cervical polyps.

 Words from the professionals

Always contact your midwife or doctor urgently if you experience vaginal bleeding so that they can decide if any further action is needed.

HORMONAL CHANGES

There are times during pregnancy when you could be forgiven for thinking that you have morphed back into a teenager with spotty skin, greasy hair and raging mood swings. And yes, as in teenagers, hormones *are* responsible for those unattractive aspects and several more besides. Here are some more symptoms caused by hormonal havoc.

Bleeding gums

Changing hormone levels cause your gums to swell and become more sensitive than normal; this can lead to bleeding gums and soreness, sometimes called pregnancy gingivitis. Some women develop little outgrowths of their gums, which occasionally bleed. These growths (known as pregnancy epulis) often appear early on in the pregnancy and usually disappear towards the end.

What can I do?

- Plaque can exacerbate the problem, so ensure you brush properly twice a day with a fluoride toothpaste, floss and use a mouthwash.

- Don't panic if your gums bleed when you brush; you need to get rid of plaque to ensure you don't develop gum disease.

Words from the professionals

Dental treatments are free on the NHS in pregnancy, so make sure you get an exemption form from your doctor or midwife and book an appointment early in your pregnancy to nip any potential problems in the bud.

Pre-eclampsia and thrombosis

There are two important disorders that can be extremely serious, even fatal, in pregnancy: pre-eclampsia and thrombosis. Read up about them so you know what signs to look out for, but don't scare yourself stupid, because your doctor and midwife will be on the lookout for them at every routine appointment. They are both uncommon.

Pre-eclampsia affects up to one in 10 pregnant women and almost always develops after 20 weeks. It usually involves high blood pressure, protein in your urine, and sometimes a smaller-than-expected baby. Often it is mild, but sometimes it can be very serious and make you or the baby unwell, necessitating early delivery. It is often detected during an antenatal appointment – this is why you always have your blood pressure measured and urine tested.

Most women have no symptoms. Sometimes intense headaches, rapid and aggressive swelling of the hands, feet and/or face, blurred vision, upper stomach ache and vomiting occur. If you develop any of these you should usually phone the hospital for their advice.

If pre-eclampsia is diagnosed you will usually be admitted to hospital. This is so that you and the baby can be monitored more carefully, and so that if either of you gets suddenly unwell, you are in a place where the right care can be given by your doctor or midwife. While the chance of this happening is small, and being stuck in hospital can be boring, it is really worthwhile listening to the advice you are being given. You may be prescribed medication to lower your blood pressure and you may need extra scans or blood tests. You may also be told you need to deliver earlier than nature was planning, as this is the only 'cure'.

Many women are offered low-dose aspirin tablets to take every day from 12 weeks of pregnancy to reduce their chances of getting pre-eclampsia. Mention this to your midwife if you think you are at increased risk of getting pre-eclampsia.

Less than two women in 100 will develop a severe form of pre-eclampsia, which might include convulsions, stroke, kidney failure, liver damage and blood clotting problems in the mother; and growth restriction, placental abruption and severe prematurity in the baby, so its risks should not be underestimated. If you want more info about pre-eclampsia visit action-on-pre-eclampsia.org.uk.

Thrombosis is the clotting of blood within a blood vessel. This blood clot can block a vein or an artery and obstructs or stops the flow of blood.

Less than two women in 1,000 develop a blood clot in a vein during pregnancy or just after birth; the risk is around five times higher than normal because blood clots and flows differently during pregnancy. Some women are more at risk because their parents or siblings have had a clot, or because they are overweight, older (which sadly is defined in this context as over 35!), less mobile, smokers or have certain medical problems – especially involving the kidneys. If you have any of these risk factors you may need to take some form of prevention against thrombosis during the pregnancy. Your midwife will ask you questions about clotting when you attend your booking appointment, and your risk of getting a clot will be reviewed if you are admitted to hospital and when you have the baby. If you have had a thrombosis before you are very likely to need extra advice during the pregnancy, so make sure your midwife and GP are aware as early as possible.

Deep vein thrombosis (DVT) is the most common type of thrombosis in pregnancy and is a blood clot that occurs in a deep vein, usually in the leg. Symptoms include pain, tenderness and swelling in the leg, and it may turn pale blue or reddish-purple in colour.

If you develop a DVT you will be given heparin to thin the blood, and you'll probably be advised to wear compression stockings to reduce the swelling and improve blood flow. You will probably need treatment for three months or even longer.

If you suspect you have a DVT you should seek immediate medical advice. It has a very dangerous complication called pulmonary embolism, when the blood clot or a piece of a blood clot breaks off and travels to the lungs where it can block one of the blood vessels. Potentially life-threatening, pulmonary embolism may cause chest pain, shortness of breath, or the coughing up of blood – if you get any of these symptoms you should get immediate medical advice, as prompt diagnosis and treatment are essential.

Tender breasts

One of the most striking aspects of pregnancy is how quickly you could give a glamour model a run for her money. For girls who struggle to fill a B cup this can be a most positive thing, but if you have fairly big breasts to start with it can be a tad alarming, and quite uncomfortable.

Hormonal activity, increased blood flow and the beginning of milk production all contribute to an increase in bust size in the first trimester, and regrettably this can have some more unwelcome side effects in the form of tenderness or discomfort.

What can I do?

Go and get yourself measured and fitted for a new non-wired bra as soon as you feel your breast size increase.

- You should get properly measured several times during your pregnancy for a non-wired bra as you may go up as much as three cup sizes.

- If you are really uncomfortable at night, try sleeping in a non-wired cotton bra.

- Some women can't bear to be touched when their breasts hurt; others find massaging them helps, so find out what works for you. Undoubtedly you'll have a willing volunteer in your partner if you opt for the latter form of relief!

- Try holding a cool damp flannel over your breasts to relieve tenderness.

Food cravings

Why we get cravings for wonderful and downright weird foodstuffs in pregnancy is a bit of a mystery, but what we do know is that they are real and most women get them to a greater or lesser degree. There's the evolutionary theory that it's just the body craving what it needs to sustain the pregnancy, or it may be triggered by your body demanding certain foods to cover nutritional deficiencies.

Some women start wanting weird combinations, such as mackerel and yoghurt, whereas others crave food they usually hate, like beetroot or jellied eels.

What can I do?

You don't need us to tell you that a diet of baked beans and ice cream is not ideal for your baby or your waistline, so our best advice is to try to follow a balanced diet.

Eat your food slowly so you don't get indigestion and heartburn, and remember that a little of what you fancy will do you good ... (unless it's inedible).

You may find this hard to believe, but craving something that is not food (such as coal) is a recognised medical disorder called pica. Munching sand, chalk, talcum powder, soap, rubber, wood or plaster isn't a great idea. If you do feel the urge to chomp a non-edible object, try to distract yourself; remove it from the house if possible and discuss it with your doctor.

Hair changes

Fluctuating hormones can play havoc with your hair: some women shed it, some women grow it, some women report glossy locks and others lanky locks, so it's difficult to predict what will happen. And it's not just the hair on your head that's affected. Pregnancy can affect your body hair as well: some find it stops growing, while some find they start developing facial hair. Unfortunately there's no way to influence what will happen to you.

What can I do?

You can wax, pluck and shave all you like, but seek advice if you want to use laser treatment or electrolysis to remove hair, as some practitioners don't encourage it. If you are using a hair removal cream, do a patch test first, because skin does become more sensitive in pregnancy.

Tackling your bikini line post 30 weeks is not a breeze! Being pregnant is the time to relax about your usual beauty rituals and concentrate on your bump, rather than your hairy bits.

Once your hormones settle down after the birth so will your hair. Don't be alarmed if it comes out in handfuls after the birth; you're very unlikely to go bald. It's just your body shedding those glossy thick locks everyone commented on while you were pregnant!

Heartburn and indigestion

Pain in the upper chest and tummy, a burning feeling or the sensation that something is stuck at the top of your tummy are all signs of heartburn or indigestion. It's not necessarily something you ate, but those dreaded hormones causing your digestive system to relax, leading to excess acid collecting in the stomach and backtracking into the gullet (oesophagus). Towards the end of your pregnancy the growing uterus puts pressure on your stomach, and this too can cause pain and discomfort in the tummy.

What can I do?

Many pregnant women swear that their best friend during pregnancy was a bottle of Gaviscon. If you are really suffering, go and see your pharmacist, and get them to recommend an over-the-counter antacid remedy suitable to take during pregnancy.

Here are some tips to avoid indigestion.

- Eat smaller meals and chew them slowly.

- If certain foods bring on an attack (spicy and greasy foods are the usual suspects), eliminate them from your diet.

- Drinking a glass of cold milk helps some women.

- Don't lie down for at least two hours after your last meal, and then try sleeping propped up on a pile of plump pillows.

Words from the professionals

Indigestion and heartburn are uncomfortable, but there's no need for you to worry: it will go away once the baby is born. Occasionally a heartburn-type sensation can be a symptom of pre-eclampsia, though, so if your indigestion is unusually severe, persistent and troublesome, seek advice.

Bad heartburn can make asthma worse, as the acid from the stomach may get into the lungs and irritate them. If you think this may be happening to you, tell your midwife or doctor.

Morning sickness

Firstly, the name 'morning sickness' is misleading because, for many women, the feeling of sickness goes on all day. Around 85% of women suffer from nausea and sickness to some degree during their pregnancy. The 'lucky' ones will feel mildly nauseous, whereas some women will physically retch and vomit all day. It tends to settle after the first trimester.

Doctors aren't 100% certain what causes it, but it's pretty likely that the fluctuation in hormone levels is to blame.

There is an evolutionary theory that it is nature's way of putting you off potentially hazardous foods. This may be true in the case of wine: many pregnant women find they can't even stand the smell of it, let alone the taste; but when you can't even keep a healthy breakfast down, the theory wears a bit thin.

If you are afflicted in the mornings, try getting up slowly and making your routine as leisurely and relaxed as possible. Leaping out of bed and snatching some toast on the hoof isn't going to help. It's also important to eat as soon as you get up, because nausea is often worse on an empty stomach.

We are all aware of the importance of a good diet even when we are not pregnant, so it can be very worrying when you feel you are not nourishing the new life growing inside you because you're living on a diet of mashed potatoes and ginger biscuits. Please don't fret about this: your baby will be able to get enough nutrients from you, however bad your diet is. To reassure yourself you only have to think about women in developing countries who have very limited access to nutritious food, and who still manage to have healthy babies, despite their restricted diets. There are many very safe medicines available to control nausea and vomiting, so you don't need to suffer in silence; if the other approaches aren't enough, talk with your doctor or midwife about suitable medication.

Vomiting in itself is not a worry, but if it is accompanied by fever or pain you should seek medical advice. It is unusual to get vomiting for the first time after 12 weeks, so if this happens again seek medical advice.

What can I do?

- Ginger is an alternative remedy that is considered effective. Try infusing a ginger root in boiling water or use ginger tea bags for a soothing hot drink. You can even nibble on ginger biscuits or suck crystallised ginger whenever you are feeling nauseous.

- Eat little and often if you can.

- Sea sickness bands can be helpful for reducing nausea. Homeopathic remedies can also help.

- Cut out things that make the problem worse – usually greasy and spicy food – and be prepared to experiment to find things that you can stomach. Bland food, such as mashed potato, white rice or bread, often does the trick.

- If you really can't face food, don't worry, but it is essential that you keep yourself hydrated; drink plenty of fluids, particularly if you are actually vomiting.

 Words from the professionals

If you vomit excessively, you could be suffering from hyperemesis gravidarum, which essentially consists of persistent vomiting, usually with weight loss, needing intravenous rehydration. Your baby will probably not be affected by this condition but you may have to be hospitalised if you become severely dehydrated. Recently more and more hospitals are offering outpatient care for this condition, so do ask. There are anti-sickness medications that you can take safely, so seek advice from your doctor or midwife if you are really suffering.

Mood swings

Pregnancy is quite tough emotionally and there's no getting away from it. You know you should be on cloud nine and super happy, but half the time you're weeping at some soppy movie on TV or wondering why you ever thought that having a baby with *him* was a good idea. Wanting to throttle your partner or cry for England is all totally normal and is a result of your raging hormones. To further compound the problem, if you are not feeling great physically, this can make you feel more vulnerable emotionally.

What can I do?

It's those damn hormones doing their worst and there's nothing you can do to prevent it happening, but there are things you can do to lift your mood.

- Talking is always good. Discuss your anger, frustrations or worries with a friend or your partner, as a trouble shared really can be a trouble halved.

- Go and see a feel-good chick flick with your mates. Cinema trips will be harder once the baby is born, so treat yourself and have a good night out with the girls.

- Even in the depths of winter the sun's watery rays can cast a little bit of sunshine on us all. Go for a walk, as it can make you feel better physically and emotionally.

- Join a pregnancy yoga class. Not only will it keep you fit and supple for labour, but it's a great stress buster too.

- Sleep, sleep and more sleep. If you are feeling good physically you'll feel better emotionally.

 Words from the professionals

There is evidence to suggest that women who are low or depressed during pregnancy have a greater chance of developing postnatal depression. If you are prone to this problem or have prolonged periods of depression during your pregnancy, do speak to your doctor, because he can refer you for counselling or prescribe something to help you.

Skin changes

Even if your teenage years were Clearasil-free, you might become a spotty mum-to-be. This is because your hormones release more sebum: an oily substance to keep the skin supple. Hormonal changes can even alter the pigmentation in your skin, causing dark patches on fair skin and light patches on dark skin.

Some women develop eczema for the first time during pregnancy, particularly over the bump, where the skin becomes very taut. Others who are already prone to the condition may have more flare-ups or find it disappears completely. To try to prevent the occurrence of eczema, keep your skin as well moisturised as possible, use very gentle soap products or get your doctor to prescribe you special emollients for the bath or shower to stop your skin drying out.

You might also notice that the area around your nipples (the areola) darkens and a dark line running down the centre of your tummy appears. This is known as the linea nigra. Moles may appear darker and you may develop skin tags anywhere on the face and body. If you are worried about any moles that start growing or changing colour during pregnancy, see your doctor to get them checked out.

The increased blood flow to the skin can give you a lovely rosy glow; it can also give you spider naevi – small clusters of tiny capillaries usually over the upper chest or arms – which are somewhat less attractive!

Given the number of changes hormones can cause in your skin, it's no surprise that it isn't a good idea to sunbathe while you're pregnant. Your skin will be more sensitive than normal, so if you are out in the sun make sure you use a high-factor sun protection.

What can I do?

The good news is that your skin normally returns to normal once the baby is born. However, there are a few things you can to do alleviate the changes.

- Review your beauty regime if your skin becomes oily and go for a medicated cleanser if you're getting unwelcome outbreaks.

- A green-coloured concealer will take the redness out of your complexion and also covers up those pesky broken veins.

- Treat yourself to a facial or a makeover to give yourself a boost.

Smell

You may find that your hormones make you incredibly sensitive to smell from virtually the moment you confirm your pregnancy. For some women, this kicks in almost immediately, and the smell of the fridge at work is so repugnant that they can't even get the milk out!

Just like morning sickness, the theory goes that you are repulsed by the smell of things which you shouldn't consume during pregnancy: so, in some cases, women can't stand the smell of beer.

What can I do?

Your sensitivity to smells may subside with your morning sickness, or it may continue throughout your pregnancy. Try these tips if you are suffering.

- Good food hygiene is common sense and if you wrap things properly in the fridge they shouldn't smell.

- Avoid crowded public transport in summer if you can: sweaty bodies in a confined area is enough to make anyone retch!

PHYSICAL EFFECTS

Breathing, walking, sleeping and thinking are all things we take for granted but they can all become tricky in pregnancy.

Breathing

We normally take breathing for granted, which is why it can be a bit worrying when you become breathless in pregnancy. Your lungs need to work harder to provide extra oxygen for you and your baby, which can make you feel breathless. Towards the end of your pregnancy the uterus might be pushing on the diaphragm (the muscle that regulates your breathing) and this will also cause breathlessness.

What can I do?

There's no need to panic if you feel breathless, but it's worth sitting down and resting if you can. It's common to feel short of breath when walking to work or going upstairs – just allow yourself more time and slow down a bit!

If you have palpitations or chest pain or an acute episode of sudden shortness of breath, do seek medical advice urgently, as it could be a sign of something more serious.

Exhaustion

It's incredibly common to feel exhausted in the early stages of pregnancy as your body works overtime to set up your baby's support systems in your uterus. Towards the end of your pregnancy, your body is carrying the equivalent of around seven bags of sugar, so it's no wonder you feel exhausted. Morning sickness, poor diet and lack of exercise can also contribute to feeling shattered.

What can I do?

- It goes without saying that you need to get as much sleep as you can. If you are still working, try to have early nights during the week and lie in at the weekends.

- Listen to your body: if it is telling you it is tired, give in and have that afternoon siesta or power nap.

- To make life as easy for yourself as you can, accept help from friends and family. How about doing your weekly supermarket shop online?

- Some light exercise can help you feel less tired.

 Words from the professionals

Exhaustion can also be a sign of anaemia, so make sure you get checked out.

Insomnia

Sometimes it's hard to sleep in pregnancy because of physical symptoms such as heartburn, backache or an overactive bladder. It could be that your baby is literally kicking you awake or you might be mentally overactive: baby anxiety has kept many a pregnant woman wide awake into the wee small hours.

What can I do?

- Avoid caffeine in the evening, as it can keep you awake and necessitate a night-time trip to the loo.

- Make yourself as comfortable as you can in bed, with comfy pillows supporting your back and your bump.

- Pop a little lavender bag under your pillow; it makes the room smell heavenly and has restful qualities.

- Don't over-stimulate your brain watching TV or using electronic devices in bed.

- Some women have strange dreams and even nightmares during pregnancy – talk to your partner or midwife to dispel any anxiety.

 Words from the professionals

If you're worried you're not getting enough sleep because of depression or anxiety, talk to your doctor or midwife. Sleeping tablets are not recommended, not least because they cross through the placenta to the baby, but talking therapies can be very helpful for some people. Some cynical people say the altered sleeping pattern is preparing you for life after the baby is born!

Baby brain

No one seems to know why pregnant women develop 'baby brain', but what we do know is that many pregnant women do seem to become extraordinarily forgetful during pregnancy. A recent study by scientists at Bradford and Leeds Universities seems to support the theory that hormones are to blame for short-term memory loss, but another study claimed that 'baby brain' is actually a myth – at least physiologically. It seems that the only explanation for any memory trouble you're having is that your pregnancy is occupying so many of your thoughts that everything else gets pushed to the side.

What can I do?
It can be frustrating and embarrassing when you keep forgetting things, so try these tips to help your memory.

- Try carrying a large diary around so that you can write down all your appointments and work meetings.

- Keep a small pocket notebook handy for lists.

Unless you do something dangerous – like drive the wrong way up a motorway – there is no need to worry if you become more absent-minded; your brain should be delivered back to you with your baby!

LEG PROBLEMS

For some reason your poor old legs can take a pasting during pregnancy. Let's stroll through a few of the most common problems.

Oedema

Swelling, or oedema, is extremely common in pregnancy: it can affect your face and hands and invariably makes its presence felt in the legs. It is caused by fluid leaking out of blood vessels with sluggish flow, and gets worse if you have been standing for long periods of time or in hot weather. Your feet may actually grow during pregnancy and not return to their original size!

What can I do?

- Invest in a pair of Crocs. Love 'em or loathe 'em, they are brilliant when you are pregnant. They are loose enough to accommodate pudgy swollen feet, and if you buy the proper ones they have 'nibbles' on the bottom to massage your soles. They are also the perfect shoes to venture into dreaded hospital bathrooms.

- Support tights are fantastic if you are on your feet all day. Granted, they are not the sexiest of fashion accessories, but they really do what it says on the packet.

- Literally put your feet up whenever you can.

- Practise foot rotation exercises when you are sitting down.

Swelling of the body can be an indication of pre-eclampsia and your doctor and midwife will be alert to the signs, so if you are worried or suddenly balloon out, get some advice as soon as you can.

Restless leg syndrome

If your legs feel as if they are tingling, burning, 'crawling' or you have an uncontrollable urge to move your legs, you may have restless leg syndrome (RLS). This affliction tends to strike at night when you are sitting down or sleeping, which makes resting or snoozing really difficult. One in five pregnant women develops RLS during pregnancy.

What can I do?
Cutting down on alcohol and caffeine helps, but hopefully you've pretty much knocked that on the head anyway.

A recent study suggested that women who took gentle/moderate exercise regularly in pregnancy were less likely to suffer from RLS, and doing gentle stretching exercises in the morning and evening will also help.

RLS can be a sign of anaemia, so do visit your doctor. If iron deficiency is detected, iron tablets will be prescribed by your doctor to alleviate your symptoms.

Varicose veins

Swollen bulging veins that may ache or itch are a common feature of pregnancy. Your hormones cause your blood vessels to relax and your body's increased blood volume and growing uterus put pressure on your veins, causing them to swell.

Varicose veins occur most commonly on the legs, but also around the anus (known as piles) and in the vaginal area (see page 76). They are partly hereditary, and being overweight, carrying twins or having many pregnancies also increase your risk of getting them.

What can I do?

- The advice is very similar to that given if you're suffering from swelling: keep your feet raised on cushions when you are resting; wear support tights during the day; and if you are on your feet all day, make sure you have regular rests, as you have a legal entitlement to do so.

- If they are hurting, you can pop an ice pack or bag of frozen peas on them to soothe the pain.

- Make sure you take regular exercise to boost your circulation.

We'd love to tell you that they go away after birth, but this is not always the case. The bad news is that unless they are causing you real pain removal is considered to be a non-essential cosmetic procedure; therefore you are not entitled to have them removed on the NHS. If you have private health insurance and a sympathetic GP you might be able to get them done on your policy for free. If you do need surgery, try to wait until you have had all your babies, as pregnancy after surgery can make new ones appear!

UP CLOSE AND PERSONAL

There are certain problems you might suffer from during pregnancy that you would prefer to keep mum about. However, pretty much anything you're going through is completely normal. Don't suffer in silence – get help if you need it.

Constipation

Pregnancy hormones relax the digestive system, causing the movement of food to slow down – so if you were prone to constipation before you became pregnant, it is likely you are going to suffer now. The pressure of the uterus on the bowels also restricts their ability to function properly, so there are two reasons why doing a number two may be problematic for you now.

What can I do?

- Drinking lots of water is a must, and a fibre-rich diet of wholemeal bread, fruit, vegetables and pulses should get things moving.

- Regular exercise such as swimming and walking can wake up a sluggish system.

- If you are prescribed iron tablets for anaemia, consider switching to different ones if they make you pass pellets like a rabbit (quite common, honestly!).

- If you are completely bunged up, you might need a mild laxative to get you going. Consult your midwife or pharmacist, as some are too strong to use in pregnancy.

Incontinence

Your pelvic floor (which supports the bladder) comes under a lot of stress during pregnancy as your uterus grows. The hormone relaxin, which makes your muscles relax in preparation for birth, can make the problem even worse. For some pregnant women the problem can be so bad that they leak when they laugh, sneeze or cough.

What can I do?

- Start doing pelvic floor exercises – also known as Kegels – ideally as soon as you discover you are pregnant (see page 108).

- Use a panty liner or pad to protect your clothes (and your dignity).

- When you go for a wee, rock back and forth slowly to make sure your bladder is completely empty.

 Words from the professionals

Giving birth can sometimes damage the pelvic floor and make it even weaker, leading to long-term incontinence problems that might require surgery. Therefore it really is of paramount importance for you to get going with those Kegel exercises. The good thing is that no one can see you doing them, so you can practise at the bus stop, in the hospital waiting room or sitting at your desk.

Piles

Probably the least favourite pregnancy symptom (and one of the most common), piles (or haemorrhoids) are like little bunches of grapes that protrude around your back passage area (that's probably the most polite way of putting it). They are caused by your hormones making the veins in that area relax, and if you're having problems with constipation, straining on the loo will exacerbate the problem further. They can itch, ache and sometimes bleed.

What can I do?

- Drink lots of water and eat fibre-rich food to keep everything moving in that department, so you don't have the extra difficulty of constipation to contend with.

- Sitting on an ice pack or frozen peas can numb the pain and soothe the area.

- Take gentle exercise regularly.

- You can ask your pharmacist to recommend an ointment to alleviate the symptoms, or, if they are really bad, you can ask your doctor to prescribe some suppositories.

Piles normally shrink back or disappear after childbirth; however, if they persist there is a medical procedure you can have. Fingers crossed they'll go of their own accord.

Stretch marks

These purple and pink lines can appear anywhere you gain weight during pregnancy, including your thighs, hips and bottom, as well as your tummy and breasts. They fade to silvery-grey in time, but once you have them they won't go away. It's difficult to know whether you will be affected: a great deal depends on your skin type and it doesn't seem to be hereditary. They can affect up to 80% of women.

What can I do?

There are many brands of cream out there that claim to help prevent stretch marks but there's no concrete evidence that any of them actually work. Cocoa butter is supposed to be effective, is cheap as chips, and smells quite nice so it might be worth giving that a go, but feel free to splurge as your budget allows. Logic says that you should probably start early, before your bump becomes too pronounced.

Thrush

You are 10 times more likely to develop thrush (also called candida) in pregnancy, because hormones affect the natural balance of bacteria in your vagina and can allow this annoying yeast to take hold.

What can I do?

- Natural yoghurt is said to contain active bacteria that can combat thrush, so you can eat it (preferably) or apply it directly to soothe your vaginal area.

- Wash carefully with unperfumed soap not more than once daily, and wear cotton knickers.

- You're probably not feeling much like having sex if you have thrush, but it can be passed on through sexual contact. If you think your partner might be affected he'll need treatment too.

- When you pass urine make sure you dry from 'front to back', not the other way – thrush lives in the back passage, and it's very easy for it to hop out into the vagina if you drag it forwards with the loo roll!

- Thrush is not dangerous for you or the baby. It only needs to be treated if it is troubling you, with an antifungal cream or pessaries. Some brands are not suitable for use in pregnancy, so ask your pharmacist or doctor to recommend or prescribe a suitable one for you.

Urination

Needing to pee more often can kick in almost as soon as you confirm your pregnancy, and annoyingly the urge often strikes in the middle of the night. Hormones are normally responsible in the early weeks, but as your pregnancy progresses your kidneys step up a gear to rid your body of excess waste products. In the third trimester the pressure on your bladder from your expanding uterus means you'll be visiting the loo more than usual as well.

If your urine is cloudy or bloody or it's painful to pee, you probably have a urinary tract infection. This can trigger premature labour, so seek medical advice if you have these symptoms. You need to provide a urine sample at every pregnancy check up. This is partly to look for signs of pre-eclampsia and partly for detecting infection.

What can I do?

- Don't restrict your fluid intake to minimise trips to the loo, as both you and your baby need plenty of liquid to keep healthy during pregnancy. You'll just have to grin and bear it!

- Avoid caffeine, particularly in the evening, as it has a diuretic effect.

- Try to empty your bladder completely when you go. Tipping your pelvis back and forth a little can help ensure you get rid of everything properly.

- Find out where the loos are when you're somewhere unfamiliar to avoid feeling desperate.

Vaginal discharge

You may experience an increase in vaginal discharge during pregnancy. It is believed that this is nature's way of protecting against infections that could travel up into your uterus, but it also happens if you have a cervical ectropion (see page 63). It may be clear, white, grey, yellow or even greenish!

Near your due date you may experience a thick show of discharge, tinged with blood, that normally indicates labour is imminent. If this happens, you should prepare yourself for the fact that you might be about to go into labour.

If the discharge changes colour, smells, or stings, mention this to your midwife. If you start leaking a watery discharge in late pregnancy this should be reported to a doctor immediately, because you might be losing amniotic fluid as a result of premature rupture of the membranes.

What can I do?
As with thrush, wash carefully with unperfumed soap and wear cotton knickers with a panty liner (not a tampon) if you feel the discharge is particularly heavy.

Vaginal varicose veins

These form in the same way as varicose veins in your legs or piles, but obviously they're in a slightly more delicate place!

What can I do?
You can buy something called a V Brace, which resembles a large pair of padded support pants. Hardly Agent Provocateur, but they do keep everything safely gathered in.

Wind

Wind has the same cause as constipation and is often related.

What can I do?

- Specific foods (such as spicy food like curry) can trigger the condition, so try to eliminate them from your diet.

- Don't overload your system with big meals – particularly late at night – and eat slowly, ensuring you chew your food thoroughly.

- Keeping active can stop wind from getting trapped in your stomach.

- There are products such as Wind-eze on the market that may relieve the symptoms of flatulence and trapped wind, but it is important that you consult a pharmacist or your midwife before you take them to check they are suitable for you.

- Some women find mints, peppermint oil or peppermint tea can alleviate symptoms.

When to seek medical help

If you are experiencing any of the symptoms below, call your maternity unit as they *may* indicate a serious problem that could threaten the health of you or your baby.

- Severe, persistent abdominal pain.
- Disturbance of vision.
- Sudden or severe swelling on your face or hands – particularly if you have a headache.
- Raging thirst and lack of urination.
- Severe vomiting accompanied by pain or fever.
- Fluid leaking from the vagina.
- Severe headache that persists for more than a few hours.
- Pain or burning on urination.
- Severe itching all over your body.
- Lack of fetal movements.
- Vaginal bleeding.
- Frequent dizzy or fainting spells.
- A heavy fall (although your baby is well cushioned in his amniotic sac, it's best to get yourself checked out if you take a tumble).

PREGNANCY PREENING

Pregnancy doesn't just affect your health; it affects the way you both look and feel, and in this section we suggest ways to make you feel more beautiful on the outside *and* on the inside.

Hair

Limp and lanky or gloriously glossy? Your hair may become luxuriously thick and fabulous or come out in handfuls, and it's notoriously difficult to predict what effect your hormones are going to have on your hair follicles. Your hair might become drier than normal or much greasier, and some women report that it changes texture too. You might also find your hair grows quicker than normal.

A trip to the hairdresser's is a great pick-me-up, and in the first trimester, when you might be feeling a bit sick and grotty, a new hairstyle or even a wash and blow dry will give you a much-needed injection of confidence. See page 110 for more on dyeing your hair.

Hands and nails

Some women find that they grow fabulous talons in pregnancy, while others find their nails become brittle and split. If you fall into the latter camp, the best advice is to keep them short, and protect them with gloves if you are doing chores such as gardening or cleaning.

If you do think your hands need a little TLC, you could treat yourself to a manicure or pedicure. It's worth remembering, however, that nail varnish is usually removed before surgeries – including Caesarean sections. During surgery, levels of oxygen in the blood are measured via a red light that passes through tissue. A device is placed on the fingertip and monitored by the anaesthetist. Nail varnish can reduce the effectiveness of the equipment.

You can also lavish your hands daily with your favourite hand cream to make them super soft and silky.

Chemical considerations

The smell of nail polish is pretty horrible even when you are not pregnant, so it's not surprising to learn that these enticing bottles of pretty coloured liquid are jam-packed with nasty chemicals. There isn't any conclusive evidence to prove that nail varnish is dangerous, but some women prefer not to take the risk and go varnish-free or use one of the increasing number of less-toxic brands – google 'natural nail polish' for online retailers.

Facial skin

You will have read earlier in this chapter that your skin can be adversely affected in pregnancy. It becomes more sensitive, can be prone to spots and can develop pigmentation marks or rashes.

Chloasma, otherwise known as 'pregnancy mask', is relatively common during pregnancy and is thought to be due to hormonal changes in the body. Chloasma is the development of darker pigmentation marks, usually on your face, and can be quite distressing to acquire. There's not a great deal that can be done for you medically, but you can use foundation or concealer to even out the skin colour, and the good news is that it usually fades within a few months of giving birth.

In terms of beauty treatments, you should avoid anything that involves chemicals (such as peels); as your skin is more sensitive, also avoid micro-dermabrasion, as you might experience adverse reactions like redness and itchiness.

If you become very spotty, check with the pharmacist before you slather your face in zit cream, because some of the stronger products on offer contain chemicals that could be harmful to your baby.

There are many beauty therapists that advertise pregnancy-specific facials and pampering. If you already have someone you use and trust, do let her know that you are pregnant, because it may affect what products she chooses.

Brilliant bosoms

Make the most of your newly acquired assets and wear a low-cut top if you fancy it; it's the perfect time to celebrate your breasts before they are put to a completely different purpose! There's no reason why you shouldn't celebrate your new curvaceous shape in all its glory.

Pregnancy is fantastic if you have small or average-sized breasts, but if you were busty to start with, it can be difficult to keep them under control. Do get yourself measured regularly. Pregnancy and maternity bras have come on leaps and bounds in recent years – some are very pretty!

Baths

There is nothing like a long, leisurely soak in the bath to soothe aching muscles and make you feel sweet-smelling and gorgeous (not to mention clean!). Some experts claim that bubble baths in pregnancy make you more prone to infection, but there isn't any hard evidence to support this.

What *is* known is that excessively hot (as opposed to warm) baths can raise your base temperature and that of your baby, and there's a slight chance that exposure to excessive heat in the uterus in the first trimester can cause neural defects. Always check the temperature of the water with your elbow. (It's also good practice for when you have the baby because this is the recommended way of doing it before you bathe him.)

If you want to properly pamper yourself, treat yourself to some yummy expensive bath oil (think of the money you're saving on wine and justify it that way!).

There are some essential oils you can drop in the bath, but this can be quite complicated. Some can't be used early in pregnancy but are safe later on (rose); some can be used throughout pregnancy and beyond (lavender); and some should be avoided at all costs (herb oils such as rosemary and thyme). Like any oils or lotions, it might be safest to stick with baby bath products.

YOUR BUMP

Like the population in general, bumps come in all different shapes and sizes. Thin people often have very prominent bumps, whereas larger people have less obvious ones; some women carry very 'high' and others 'low'; and some tend to carry out front, whereas other women go 'wide' and carry on the hip area. The shape and size of your bump depends on the following factors:

- the size of your baby and placenta

- the amount of weight you gain

- your height and general posture

- the strength of your tummy muscles (if they are strong your bump will initially be less noticeable; in subsequent pregnancies women often show earlier, as their muscles are not as strong as they were)

- the amount of amniotic fluid

- the position of the baby in the final trimester

- the number of babies you are carrying.

Most women don't show until they are at least 12 weeks. From this point your uterus begins to push out beyond your pubic bone and, depending on your weight, size and strength of your abs, your bump will make itself known to the world.

There are heaps of oils, lotions and potions that are specially developed for use in pregnancy, and it is very important that you check the provenance of anything you use on your body, because certain essential oils can be very harmful. **Never** massage them directly on the skin.

If in doubt, you can always resort to baby oils and lotions: if they are safe enough to use on a newborn, they will be fine for you to use.

While many women (and their partners) love their bodies when pregnant, there are some of you that won't enjoy having a bump, massive boobs or the other wobbly bits that you may acquire. Don't worry if you have feelings like this; it is more common than you think. Your body is doing an amazing thing – instead of having negative thoughts, try and focus on what you are achieving right now.

One of the oddest things about being pregnant is that as soon as you have a sizeable bump it suddenly becomes public property, and strangers feel totally at ease with touching your tummy. This can be most disconcerting, particularly the first time it happens – and if you are shy you will probably find this intrusion torturous. How you deal with it depends greatly on your mood; people are generally well meaning and don't want to freak you out, but if you really hate it you might just have to murmur, 'Excuse me,' and make a swift exit!

You might feel a bit terrified having read about the myriad ailments that you can experience during pregnancy, but don't panic! Pregnancy does bring some odd, unpleasant, uncomfortable and even mildly amusing side effects, but most are normal and your body will adjust to these changes. Always seek medical advice if you are concerned about any symptoms or side effects. Never feel embarrassed to ask for help.

4

My lifestyle and healthy eating

In this chapter we look at your lifestyle and how you might have to adapt it now that you are pregnant. We give you the latest information so you can make informed choices.

ALCOHOL

The Department of Health advises pregnant women to abstain from alcohol completely during pregnancy. This is not based on any evidence proving that small amounts of alcohol in pregnancy are harmful, but as doctors can't be *certain* that it doesn't have a detrimental effect on the baby, they are playing it safe and recommending you don't drink at all.

The National Institute for Health and Care Excellence (NICE) gives slightly more relaxed advice, recommending that women abstain from alcohol in the first trimester and then stick to the guideline of **no more than one or two units a week** after that.

The facts

We do know that alcohol passes from a woman's blood stream into the baby's through the placenta, and that the baby's liver and brain are very immature, so excessive drinking is very likely to harm your baby. This includes binge drinking – more than 7.5 units on one occasion. Women who drink more than six units a day have babies who are at significant risk of developing fetal alcohol syndrome, a condition that causes facial deformities, restricted growth, and learning and behavioural difficulties.

If you drink heavily in pregnancy you are also more likely to have a miscarriage in the first trimester; suffer a stillbirth; have a low-weight baby; and have a baby prone to illness.

Bear in mind that you would have to be drinking three very large glasses of wine every day to put your baby at risk of fetal alcohol syndrome, so don't scare yourself unnecessarily if you have the odd one or two in your pregnancy, or if you had a drink before you knew you were pregnant.

If you are usually a heavy drinker, tell your midwife so she can provide you with the support and advice you need to reduce your alcohol intake and monitor your baby closely.

Your choice

We cannot tell you whether you should drink or not; but we can give you the information so that you can make an informed decision.

You probably know by now that the riskiest time in terms of the baby's development and possibility of miscarriage is the first trimester, so many women choose to abstain during that period and then have the odd tipple after that.

A survey by the charity Tommy's revealed that 40% of women in the UK drank in pregnancy and that 28% drank more than the previously recommended two units a week.

There is plenty of research on this topic, and while there is conclusive evidence that heavy drinking will have a detrimental effect on your baby, there doesn't seem to be any hard evidence proving that the odd drink will do your baby any harm.

If you do want to give up or cut down on alcohol, consider these alternatives.

- Switch to low-alcohol or alcohol-free versions of beer or cider. Served chilled in the summer they can be as refreshing as the real thing.

- Many companies specialise in alcohol-free wines. www.alcoholfree.co.uk has a big selection, including mixed cases, so you can try them all and find your favourite.

- If you are pregnant in the winter, there are some nice mulled drinks and teas that are alcohol-free and quite warming for the body and soul.

Know your limits

If you do decide to enjoy the odd tipple during your pregnancy, it's essential that you know how many units you are having each time. Measures are definitely getting larger, so study the table on the following page to check that you are not consuming more units than you intend. You also need to take into account the strength of the wine: there is definitely a trend for more 'powerful' wines from Chile, South Africa and the USA, so check the alcohol by volume (ABV) on the back of the bottle before you quaff.

Wine	ABV 12%	ABV 14%
Small (125ml) glass of wine	1.5 units	1.75 units
Standard (175ml) glass of wine	2.1 units	2.45 units
Large (250ml) glass of wine	3 units	3.5 units

From this table you can see that you are exceeding your weekly unit allowance just by drinking one standard glass of wine, and that gets even higher if the wine is strong.

Drink	Units
330ml bottle of 5% strength lager	1.7
Pint of 5% strength lager	2.8
25ml of spirit	1
35ml of spirit (usual pub measure)	1.4
Double (50ml) measure of spirit	2

Stick to one bottle of beer or a pub measure of spirit and a mixer to stay on the safe side.

 Words from the professionals

In Chapter 1 we mentioned that if you went out and drank alcohol before you knew you were pregnant (even if you exceeded six units in one sitting) it is unlikely that you have done your baby any lasting damage. It is prolonged heavy drinking and binge drinking in pregnancy that does the harm. If you are having trouble giving up or cutting down, do seek help from your GP or midwife, who can refer you for specialist help.

SMOKING

If you didn't manage to stop smoking before you conceived, once your pregnancy is confirmed you should make every effort to quit for the sake of your baby. Take a look at the risks below: if they don't convince you to quit – or at the very least, cut down drastically – nothing will.

- According to research by the Health Education Authority, if you smoke during your pregnancy your risk of miscarriage increases by around 25%.

- You have a 50% increased risk of stillbirth if you smoke throughout your pregnancy, but if you quit during the first trimester your risk drops to the same as a non-smoker.

- Latest health figures show that babies born to smokers are on average 8oz lighter than babies born to non-smokers. Canadian research also shows they are also more likely to become obese teenagers.

- Smoking has been shown to increase the chance of birth defects such as a cleft palate.

- You're more likely to suffer a placental abruption if you smoke (see page 62).

- Babies born to smokers are more likely to be born prematurely at any time from 24 to 37 weeks.

- Your baby is more likely to have respiratory problems (such as asthma and chest infections) after birth.

- According to The Foundation for the Study of Infant Deaths, if you smoke one to nine cigarettes a day during pregnancy, you are four times more likely to have a baby die as a result of cot death than a non-smoker.

- A leading reproduction biologist has recently discovered that smoking in pregnancy can reduce your baby boy's sperm count and affect his future fertility.

Stubbing out the habit

It isn't always easy to give up smoking: according to ASH (Action on Smoking & Health), in certain areas of the UK as many as 33% of pregnant women continue to smoke. However, it can be paramount to the health of your baby that you try to quit. If you want to give up, make sure you see your GP or ask your midwife to put you in touch with a health professional who can help you safely quit for good. You can also check out the NHS website at www.nhs.uk/smokefree, or call the NHS smoking pregnancy helpline on 0800 123 1044. You can use any of the cigarette substitutes such as gums or patches.

Sometimes your body gives you the helping hand you need to quit: many women who were committed smokers pre-pregnancy found it quite easy to stop in the first trimester, because they were so queasy and sick that the last thing in the world they wanted was a ciggie. However, quitting cold turkey can also leave both you and your baby stressed out, so make sure you wean yourself down to a bare minimum as soon as possible, and then aim to quit completely as you adjust. Research is currently underway to see if exercise can help women to quit. E-cigarettes are also not safe in pregnancy.

 Words from the professionals

If your partner smokes, encourage him to give up too. Not only can you support each other, but your home will be smoke-free, making it a much safer environment for your newborn. Passive smoking, including toxins from his hair and body, are dangerous for you and the baby.

DRUGS

Although it's fairly obvious that illegal recreational drugs will be harmful to your baby, you also need to realise that if you take a regular prescription drug you may need to change your dosage, and even if you have a simple headache you will need to reconsider the type of painkiller you might normally reach for.

Prescription drugs

If you have a chronic or long-term condition that requires regular medication, ideally you would have discussed the condition and its treatment with your GP, the doctor you see at the hospital or an obstetrician before you conceived. Assuming you didn't quite get round to it, then you must tell your GP that you are pregnant as soon as it's confirmed, in case your medication needs to be changed or the dosage needs to be altered. Do not stop taking prescription drugs without seeking medical advice first. If you are advised to start on a prescription drug while pregnant, always remind the prescriber that you are pregnant – many drugs are safe, including, for example, most antibiotics.

Over-the-counter drugs

Pregnant women should avoid unnecessary over-the-counter medicines and drugs that you normally buy from the chemist or pharmacy. If you do buy over-the-counter drugs, you must first check with the pharmacist that they are safe to take in pregnancy: they are trained to know what is safe to take. If you have a pain that will not go away, you can take paracetamol as long as you stick to the recommended dose, and if you suffer from heartburn, a common pregnancy ailment, Gaviscon is perfectly safe to swig in moderation.

Remember it's not just products you take orally that could be risky: some creams you put on your skin could also harm your baby, so read the instructions of any product carefully before you use it. If it does not clearly state that it is safe to use in pregnancy, make sure that you ask a pharmacist, your GP, midwife, or call NHS 111 before you use it.

Homeopathic drugs

Homeopathy can play a very useful part in pregnancy as *most* of the remedies are safe to use (although not all). If you buy anything homeopathic over the counter and there isn't a qualified homeopath to advise you, do check with your midwife before you take it, because some 'natural' remedies do carry risks and won't have been carefully scrutinised for safety in the same way as conventional medicines. You need to remember that even though something is herbal, it might still be harmful. For example, essential oils can be very dangerous in pregnancy, so double-check everything before you use it.

Illegal drugs

If you continue to take recreational drugs once you know you are pregnant, you will undoubtedly put your health and that of your baby at risk.

There is plenty of research to show that taking illegal drugs in pregnancy is a bad idea. Reasons why you should stop before you conceive, or, failing that, as soon as your pregnancy is confirmed include:

- fetal growth restriction and low birth weight
- heart problems and congenital deformities
- increased risk of stillbirth
- miscarriage, early labour or placental abruption.

If you were using drugs on a one-off or occasional basis before you knew you were pregnant, do mention it to your doctor or midwife in case they want to run any additional antenatal checks. They won't judge you and it's best that they have a clear picture of your health and lifestyle. If you have an addiction to drugs, we cannot stress enough the need for you to seek professional help immediately to minimise the risks to you and your baby. If you want to speak to someone in confidence you can always call the National Drugs Helpline (0800 77 66 00), and it will put you in touch with people or organisations that can help you.

CAFFEINE

You'd think, with all that abstinence, you'd be allowed to stick your feet up and enjoy a cuppa whenever you felt like it, but it's a good idea to also keep an eye on your caffeine intake. Too much caffeine during pregnancy can cause low birth weight in babies. There have also been some studies indicating that excessive caffeine consumption can lead to miscarriage. There's not only the health of your baby to consider: excessive caffeine intake can also trigger or worsen a range of general health problems in the mother, such as insomnia, headaches, high blood pressure and dehydration, so think before you drink!

The Department of Health advises **200 micrograms of caffeine** a day as the safe limit for consumption during pregnancy. That's just two mugs of instant coffee or even less if the coffee is strong. Caffeine is also found in lesser amounts in tea, cola, chocolate and some medicines.

How much caffeine does it contain?

- Mug of instant coffee = 100mg
- Mug of filter or ground coffee = 140mg
- Mug of tea = 75mg
- Can of cola = up to 40mg
- Can of energy drink = 80mg–175mg
- 50g bar of plain chocolate = about 50mg
- 50g bar of milk chocolate = about 25mg

Here are a few tips to help you live without your caffeine fix.

- Switch to decaf versions of your favourite hot drinks.
- Try fruit teas: they have no caffeine in them and can be quite refreshing served hot or iced.
- Switch to caffeine-free cola.
- Try having a glass of water instead.

Finally, if you do exceed the safe limit occasionally, don't beat yourself up about it; it's unlikely to do your baby any damage as long as it's an occasional thing.

X-rays

The risk from diagnostic X-rays is extremely low, and, usually, if you are advised to have an X-ray this will be because the benefits to you (and therefore the baby) of helping to make a diagnosis vastly outweigh any tiny worries. For example, a chest X-ray has the same amount of radiation as 10 days of background radiation in the general atmosphere, or a one-way flight from the UK to New York. If it's essential to have one in your pregnancy, the radiographer will still do everything she can to protect your unborn child. If an X-ray is non-urgent, it can probably wait until your baby is born. If you need an X-ray at the dentist's he will provide a special protective apron to cover your bump.

Words from the professionals

It is best to avoid drinking herbal teas while you're pregnant, especially ones containing unfamiliar ingredients such as ginseng or black cohosh. The active ingredients in these can cross the placenta with unknown consequences. Raspberry leaf tea is thought to be a uterine stimulant, meaning it could be linked with the onset of labour, so it's best avoided until the last few weeks of pregnancy (see page 211).

FOOD

In pregnancy your immune system is suppressed, which means you're more likely to get food poisoning. As well as making you sick this could have harmful effects on your baby. If you suspect you have contracted anything potentially dangerous from food you should contact your GP as soon as possible, as he may be able to treat you quickly and prevent the infection spreading to your baby.

Before we start ...

In this section we go through the reasons why some foods aren't recommended during pregnancy, but you mustn't get too hung up about what you ate before you knew you were pregnant, or worry about an occasional mistake during pregnancy: normally, the chances of your baby being harmed are minute. We've included the most commonly avoided foods here, but it's not a definitive list.

Meat

Undercooked or raw meat can harbour several types of food poisoning: toxoplasmosis, salmonella, campylobacter and E. coli.

The risk of getting toxoplasmosis while you're pregnant is very low in the UK. Women with the infection normally get flu-like symptoms, such as a high temperature and aching limbs – but if contracted by an unborn child it can cause miscarriage, stillbirth or serious complications including brain damage and blindness.

If you suspect you contracted toxoplasmosis in the three months prior to pregnancy or during pregnancy itself, visit your doctor as soon as possible.

 Words from the professionals

The toxoplasma parasite can also be found in cat poo, so be particularly careful if you have to handle this. Ideally, delegate changing the litter tray to someone else. Otherwise, wear gloves and wash your hands thoroughly afterwards. The same precautions should be taken when gardening.

How to prevent food poisoning from meat:

- ensure all meat products are well cooked, particularly poultry and barbecue items such as steak, sausages and burgers
- heat ready-meals or convenience food thoroughly, ensuring they are hot all the way through
- pay attention to food hygiene – cover raw meat and store it away from other foods. Remember to wash your hands and any cooking utensils after handling raw meat.

Cheese

Cheese is a fantastic food to eat in pregnancy because it is a good source of protein and calcium. However, you should not eat soft cheeses such as Camembert or Brie; blue-veined cheeses such as soft Danish Blue or Dolcelatte; or soft cheeses such as mozzarella or feta if they are made from unpasteurised milk. This is because these soft cheeses are more susceptible to bacterial growth such as listeria – a bacteria which can cause an infection called listeriosis.

Check the labelling on cheeses before you buy, as quite a few are made with unpasteurised milk, though you only need to worry about the soft ones: hard unpasteurised cheese, such as parmesan, is considered safe.

Listeriosis is an incredibly rare disease, affecting between 20 and 30 pregnant women in the UK each year. However, it is estimated that during pregnancy you are 15 to 20 times more likely to become infected. It causes mild flu-like symptoms in healthy adults but can lead to serious illnesses such as meningitis, pneumonia, jaundice, premature birth or even death in an unborn baby. If you contract listeriosis in pregnancy you will be given antibiotics, as will your newborn if he is affected.

Cheeses you should avoid:

- **mould-ripened soft unpasteurised cheeses:** Brie, Blue Brie, Camembert, Chaumes, Chèvre (goat's cheese with a white rind), Pont l'Eveque, Taleggio, Vacherin
- **blue-veined cheeses:** Bleu d'Auvergne, Cambazola, Danish Blue, Dolcelatte, Gorgonzola, Roquefort, Shropshire Blue, Tomme
- **soft, unpasteurised cheeses:** goat and sheep's cheeses.

Cheeses you can safely eat:

- **hard cheeses:** Babybel, Caerphilly, Cheddar, Cheshire, Derby, Double Gloucester, Edam, Emmenthal, Gouda, Gruyère, Havarti, Jarlsberg, Lancashire, Manchego, Parmesan, pecorino (hard), Provolone, Red Leicester

- **soft cheeses (provided they are made from pasteurised milk):**
  Boursin, cottage cheese, cream cheese (eg Philadelphia), mascarpone, mozzarella, processed cheeses (eg Dairylea), quark, ricotta, feta.

If you can't live without your blue or soft cheeses, cooking them thoroughly will destroy the bacteria. So if you fancy a goat's cheese and Parma ham pizza, Brie in breadcrumbs, or Stilton soup, as long as you serve them piping hot there should be no risk to you or your baby.

Eggs

Undercooked eggs and poultry may contain salmonella – a bacterium that causes very severe food poisoning. If you contract salmonella while you are pregnant it won't pass directly to your baby as it doesn't cross the placenta. However, it can cause severe dehydration that can lead to complications and possible hospitalisation.

In 2016, the guidelines for eating runny yolks or partially cooked eggs during pregnancy changed. Now, if the eggs are produced under British Lion code (which 90% of UK eggs are) and have the lion stamp on, they are ok to serve runny. However, do be aware that imported eggs may still pose a risk, as do eggs from birds other than hens.

Foods containing egg you may want to avoid:

- home-made ice cream
- fresh hollandaise sauce
- fresh mayonnaise
- certain uncooked puddings such as home-made chocolate mousse and tiramisu.

Foods containing egg that you can eat safely:

- Shop-bought versions of all of the above should be fine because they will have been made with pasteurised eggs – ie heated to a point where the bacteria are destroyed. Baked products containing eggs, such as cakes and biscuits, are also safe.

 Words from the professionals

Not all bacteria are harmful: those probiotic yoghurts and drinks that contain 'friendly' bacteria are perfectly safe in pregnancy, as are other yoghurts and sour cream.

Ice cream

You can still eat ice cream while you are pregnant, but only shop-bought varieties: not soft ice cream (like a Mr Whippy). Soft ice cream that comes from a machine is kept at a higher temperature and there is a danger that the machine could also be harbouring germs. So if you get the urge for an ice cream when you are out and about, stick to a tub.

Liver

In the 1960s and 1970s pregnant women were encouraged to eat buckets of liver, and as it was a fairly cheap form of protein they dutifully obliged. These days, due to changes in the way animals are fed, liver contains high levels of vitamin A, which can cause birth defects.

Official guidance is to avoid all liver products, including liver pâté and sausage, but please don't worry if you ate some before you knew you were pregnant; it's very unlikely to have caused any problems.

 Words from the professionals

Cod liver oil tablets also contain vitamin A, so stop taking them as soon as you know you are pregnant, to be on the safe side.

Milk

Most milk products you find in the shops are pasteurised so are safe to consume (unpasteurised milk is normally only found in specialist shops or online), but if you have an intolerance to dairy and usually drink goat's or sheep's milk, you need to check before you buy as they may be unpasteurised.

Fish

Fish is an excellent source of protein and essential vitamins and minerals when you're pregnant; oily fish (eg salmon) also supplies long-chain omega 3 fatty acids which are important for your baby's brain and eye development. However, there are some precautions you should take.

Shellfish

It is sensible to avoid raw or undercooked shellfish, such as mussels, oysters and prawns, because they harbour salmonella and another, rather wonderfully named, germ: campylobacter.

You can eat cooked shellfish as long as you are satisfied it has been cooked properly, but it's probably best to avoid it at a buffet when you don't know how long it has been hanging around. It's also advisable to give fish stalls a miss unless you are sure of the standards of hygiene and quality of the food.

Raw fish

The Food Standards Agency's (FSA) advice on eating fish such as smoked salmon, mackerel and trout is that the risks are negligible, but as it is smoked rather than cooked it is classified as partially raw. If you can't live without it you're probably best buying it pre-packaged from a reputable supermarket, refrigerating it and eating it within the sell-by period.

Supermarket sushi is considered to be safe because it is normally frozen beforehand, which will kill any parasites. If you are making it at home, freeze it for 24 hours before consumption, and if you are eating it at a restaurant do check that it has been frozen before you tuck in.

Oily fish

Although oily fish, such as salmon, trout, sardines and mackerel, are very nutritious, they have also been found to contain traces of pollutants. So that you and your baby can benefit from the omega 3s without taking on risks from these pollutants, the FSA advises pregnant women to eat one or two portions of fish a week, including one meal of oily fish, but not to have oily fish more than twice a week.

Fish with high mercury content

Shark, swordfish and marlin may contain high levels of mercury – which has been shown to damage a baby's nervous system – so you should not eat these at all.

Tuna has also been found to contain traces of mercury, but at much lower levels, so the FSA advises pregnant women to have no more than two fresh tuna steaks or four cans of tuna a week.

Fresh pâté

There's a tiny risk of listeria in fresh pâtés, which is why official advice warns against eating even the vegetable varieties. If you can't live without it, pâtés in vacuum packs or tins are considered to be safe, but you should avoid liver pâté entirely because of the vitamin A risk.

Nuts

The latest advice from the Department of Health is that eating peanuts during pregnancy is not putting your baby at risk of developing a peanut allergy – indeed, there is some evidence to show that eating peanuts during pregnancy might protect your baby from developing such an allergy.

In the past, women with a family history of allergies were advised to avoid eating peanuts while they were pregnant. However, in 2009, the guidelines were updated and you can enjoy peanuts as part of a healthy balanced diet. If you have any worries about peanuts or other nuts talk to your midwife or doctor.

Bagged salads

You are advised to re-wash salads that have been washed and bagged, as bugs can breed in the bags in the chiller cabinet. It goes without saying that you should also wash all vegetables and salads thoroughly to remove any traces of dirt, as toxoplasmosis is transmitted through soil.

Barbecues and buffets

We've already stressed that undercooked meat is a breeding ground for bacteria, so ensure that anything you eat from the barbecue is not only properly cooked but also fresh, as bacteria can breed on food that has been left uncovered in a warm place.

If you go on a picnic, make sure that you put plenty of those ice blocks in your cool bag, place the bag in a shady spot before you eat, and don't leave it festering in the hot sun for hours while you snack. If you are at a party and suspect the food has been hanging around for a while, stick to hot food if possible and avoid prawns and cold meat platters.

Deli foods/takeaways/restaurants

Don't buy sandwiches from a deli where all the sandwich fillings look a bit tired and crusty: chances are they have probably been in the shop too long.

Don't buy food from market stalls (even from farmers' markets) if it is sitting around in the sun all day with no refrigeration.

The rule of thumb is that if something is freshly cooked and hot it should be fine, and if you did buy a slice of cold quiche from the local deli and are a bit worried about it, a blast in the oven for 15 minutes should certainly kill off any harmful bugs.

Just remember: if you want to eliminate any risk of food poisoning or contamination you'd never eat out during your pregnancy, but that's not realistic or feasible, so it's best to use common sense and follow your instincts.

Eating on holiday

If you go abroad while you are pregnant, it can be very difficult to control what you eat. It can be tricky if you are staying in a hotel that operates a buffet service at lunch or dinner; the best advice is to stick to hot food whenever possible, as in warm climates cold buffets are a breeding ground for bugs. If you can, eat food you know is freshly cooked to order, like crêpes or pizza. Sometimes it's a good idea to eat popular local food because it's more likely to be made fresh/ have a quicker turnaround than some obscure Westernised dish on the menu.

HEALTHY EATING

You don't need to go on a special diet when pregnant – just make sure it's balanced, with plenty of variety. A recent study indicated that pregnant women who ate junk food were more likely to have offspring with a sweet tooth, and another recent survey showed that children born to mothers who ate lots of junk food were more likely to suffer health problems such as heart disease and diabetes in later life, so it makes sense to adopt a healthy diet when you are pregnant.

Here's a quick summary of the foods you should be eating in pregnancy and the reasons why they are beneficial to you and your baby.

Eat regularly

It's important to eat three balanced meals a day – with a combination of food groups at each – to keep your blood sugar levels steady and to cope with the demands that pregnancy puts on your body. You may also have to top that up with healthy snacks to boost flagging energy levels. Ideal snacks to keep in your drawer or bag include bags of dried or fresh fruit, carrot or celery sticks and crispbreads or rice cakes.

Artificial sweeteners, although not ideal, are safe to have in pregnancy in moderation. Low-fat yogurts, for example, provide you with a good source of calcium and can help you watch your weight. You should try to avoid low-calorie fizzy drinks, sweets, etc as they don't contain any nutrients that will help you or your baby.

Drink lots (of water)

It's really important to keep yourself well hydrated when you are pregnant, so make sure you drink lots of fluid. Water is the healthiest choice, and it's a good idea to keep a small bottle of it with you at all times in case you get stuck travelling or in a meeting. You can supplement it throughout the day with teas, juices, milk and smoothies, but keep an eye on your caffeine levels and watch the sugar in some squashes and fruit juices, as they can be empty calories.

Fruit and vegetables

You're probably well aware that you should be aiming to eat five portions of fruit and vegetables a day, and that they can be fresh, dried, frozen or tinned.

If you'd admit to not being a regular fruit and vegetable eater, look for simple ways of sneaking them into your day. Maybe you could have sliced banana on your breakfast cereal or take dried apricots into work for a snack. Tomato-based sauces are great with pasta, and you can also purée other vegetables into them to get the nutritional benefits without them tasting overly veggie. (You'll get very adept at that at baby's weaning time too!) Eating lots of fruit and vegetables also keeps your system moving as they are full of fibre, and that's important because pregnant women are prone to constipation.

Food safety

To minimise the risk of getting food poisoning during your pregnancy, follow the simple steps below.

- Keep your kitchen clean.
- Wash your hands thoroughly before and after handling food.
- Wash fruit and vegetables properly.
- Defrost frozen food thoroughly, preferably in the fridge.
- Store raw and cooked food on different shelves in the fridge. Raw food should be kept towards the bottom as it is colder there, and also so it can't drip juice or blood onto the food below it.
- Cover food in the fridge.
- Make sure the fridge and freezer are at the correct temperature: 0–4°C for fridges and -18°C for freezers.
- Chill or freeze food as soon as you get home. If you buy food in your lunch hour, store it in the fridge at work; don't leave it by your desk.
- Have separate chopping boards for raw foods, meat and fish.
- Eat food within the sell-by date.
- Keep pets out of the kitchen if possible and definitely off the work surfaces.

Protein

Protein is very important to keep you fit and healthy and plays an important role in the development of your baby, so you need to ensure that you have plenty in your diet.

Protein-rich foods include lean white and red meat, fish (aim for two portions a week), eggs, nuts and pulses. Protein-rich foods are also rich sources of iron – another vital nutrient for your developing baby.

Dairy

Dairy products such as cheese, milk and yoghurt are great sources of calcium, which is important in the development of your baby's teeth and bones. You don't need to eat any more than usual in pregnancy, though: the recommended amount for women is 700 micrograms a day, which is a glass of milk (230mg), a pot of yoghurt (225mg) and a matchbox-sized piece of cheese (288mg).

Starchy carbohydrates

A balanced diet should include starch in the form of bread, rice, pasta or potatoes. You should try to include a portion at each mealtime, and preferably opt for wholegrain versions, as they are a better source of fibre and contain more nutrients.

Vitamins and minerals

Having covered the main food groups you should be eating, you also need to address whether your intake of vitamins and minerals is sufficient to meet the needs of you and your growing baby and decide whether you need to take additional supplements.

Iron

Iron is important for healthy blood and, as you also need to keep your baby well supplied during pregnancy, it's important to eat some of the following: fortified breakfast cereals (check for iron on the list of ingredients), meat, poultry, fish, peas, beans, lentils, green vegetables and bread. Your blood will be checked during your antenatal appointments, as anaemia is common in pregnancy, so it's worth trying to follow an iron-rich diet (anything to avoid those constipation-inducing iron tablets!). See page 57 for more on anaemia. If you do become anaemic, then iron supplements are very helpful (see page 58).

Vitamin D

Vitamin D ensures your baby's bones develop properly and boosts the content of your breast milk, which is already in production during pregnancy. Vitamin D isn't found in many foods; oily fish is an excellent source and it's found in smaller amounts in margarine and eggs. Sunlight is the greatest provider of vitamin D: dark-skinned women and those who cover their skin or don't go outside often are more at risk of vitamin D deficiency, as are those who wear strong sun block. The FSA recommends that pregnant women take a 10 microgram vitamin D supplement daily, from when they are pregnant through to breastfeeding.

Calcium

Calcium is important for the development of your baby's teeth and bones. If you are not keen on dairy products, other good sources include canned sardines. You can also get smaller amounts of calcium from wholemeal bread, baked beans, nuts (such as almonds) and green vegetables (such as broccoli). Certain cereals, juices, soy products and tofu are fortified with calcium, so do check the labels of these products when you buy them.

Latest evidence shows that supplements of calcium and extra vitamin D can lower the chance of getting pre-eclampsia; so talk with your doctor if you think you might benefit from this.

Folic acid
Women planning on becoming pregnant are advised to take 400 micrograms of folic acid as soon as they start trying for a baby until week 12 of pregnancy. Folic acid has been shown to reduce the chance of your baby developing a neural tube defect such as spina bifida. It is advisable to take this supplement and eat a diet rich in folates. Folate-rich foods include green vegetables, brown rice and fortified bread and cereals.

Omega 3: essential fatty acids
Long-chain omega 3s are thought to boost your baby's brain and eyesight development. Oily fish is the best source: mackerel, sardines, kippers, salmon or fresh tuna. Some nuts and seeds also contain omega 3s but not the long-chain type found in oily fish. There is no evidence that taking either a fish oil or omega 3 supplement is helpful in pregnancy, but many women do. See page 96 for recommendations on limiting oily fish intake during pregnancy.

Antenatal supplements

The Department of Health guidelines recommend that all women take 400 micrograms of folic acid before pregnancy and for the first 12 weeks and 10 micrograms of vitamin D throughout pregnancy and until the end of breastfeeding.

You should get all the other nutrients you need from the food that you eat, so if you are following a healthy diet like the one outlined in this book you will not need to take any other extra supplements.

If you do decide to take other supplements as well, make sure you buy a supplement developed specifically for pregnancy.

Some vitamins can be quite expensive, but bear in mind that supermarket and chemist own-brand labels will be just as good as those in fancy bottles, and if you are on benefits the government's Healthy Start programme (www.healthystart.nhs.uk) will provide them for free, so if you think you are eligible speak to your midwife.

If you take a mix of supplements, rather than a single pregnancy-specific dose, do ensure that you are not exceeding the recommended daily allowance (RDA) of anything (the RDA will be given on the bottle), as it could be harmful to your baby. Vitamin A can be harmful, so should not be taken.

WEIGHT GAIN

The well-worn cliché, 'I'm eating for two', is sadly a myth. You actually only need an extra 200 calories a day (max) to cope with the demands of pregnancy, and that's only in the third trimester.

Your weight will not be monitored throughout your pregnancy unless you are underweight or overweight or have certain medical conditions in which weight loss (eg Crohn's disease) or gain (heart disease) might indicate a problem. At your initial booking appointment your midwife will weigh you and work out your BMI (body mass index). This is your weight in kilograms divided by your height in metres squared: normal is 19–25; underweight is less than 19; and the more your BMI is over 25, the more obese you are. Being overweight or seriously underweight can be a cause for concern for you and your baby.

The Royal College of Obstetrics and Gynaecologists (RCOG) guideline, 'Care of Women with Obesity in Pregnancy', lists a depressingly long list of serious adverse outcomes that occur more frequently in obese pregnant women, and strongly encourages weight loss before conception, and healthy eating and appropriate exercise during pregnancy to minimise weight gain. These outcomes can include miscarriage, congenital anomaly in the baby, blood clots, gestational diabetes, pre-eclampsia, difficult labour and delivery, post-partum haemorrhage, stillbirth, neonatal death, wound infection and Caesarean section. You are also more prone to varicose veins, heartburn and breathlessness. Quite a scary list, right? So, for both your sakes, spend some time maintaining a healthy diet.

Be careful not to go the other way, though. Only restrict your calorie intake or diet during pregnancy under strict guidance from a doctor – if you are overweight a diet may be advised, but you will be supported and monitored. You are *supposed* to gain weight in pregnancy; after all, you have a growing baby and placenta to support. The box below shows the average distribution of weight gained during pregnancy.

Average distribution of pregnancy weight gain

- Baby: 7.5lb (3.4kg)
- Placenta: 1.5lb (0.68kg)
- Extra fluid: 3lb (1.36kg)
- Increased blood: 2.5lb (1.25kg)
- Amniotic fluid: 1.5lb (0.68kg)
- Uterus: 2lb (0.9kg)
- Fat deposits: 7lb (3.18kg)
- Breasts: 1lb (0.5kg)

Total weight gain: 26lb (12kg)

How much weight should I gain?

In an ideal world you should be your ideal weight before you conceive; many overweight women are advised to lose weight before they become pregnant so they don't encounter the types of problems outlined on page 101. If you are seriously underweight you may need to see a doctor to look into why this might be.

Both gaining too much or too little weight during pregnancy can cause problems for your baby, and too much weight gain can also cause health problems and high blood pressure for you. How much weight you should gain will relate to your body mass index, which will be measured at your initial booking appointment. Healthcare proefssionals can then advise you of ideal weight increases in line with your personal BMI.

As a rough guide, you can expect to put on between 10kg and 12.5kg (22lb and 28lb) during your pregnancy, with most of it being gained after 20 weeks. If you are overweight, you should seek advice from your midwife about pregnancy weight gain. Your midwife will be able to offer guidance to ensure you don't gain too much weight.

Gestational diabetes (GDM)

Diabetes occurs when the body doesn't make enough of the hormone insulin or when the body is resistant to the effects of insulin, resulting in high levels of blood sugar. Gestational diabetes is the same condition but is brought on by pregnancy. In pregnancy you need to make twice as much insulin to sustain both you and the baby, and many women are unable to do so. This allows blood sugar levels to rise and gestational diabetes develops. With gestational diabetes your antenatal care will usually be transferred into a specialist pregnancy diabetes clinic, with support from a dietician, diabetes nurse specialist and midwife.

Units will test either all or just some women for GDM at around 26 to 28 weeks' gestation, so ask your midwife if you need a test. NICE recommends screening if:

- your BMI is greater than 30
- there is diabetes in a first-degree relative
- a previous baby weighed more than 4.5kg at birth
- your ethnic origin is Afro-Caribbean, Asian or Middle-Eastern
- you are more than 30 years old.

Healthy eating and exercise often keeps your blood sugar levels under control, but you may need tablets or insulin injections if you develop this condition. You must also make sure you get a check-up when the baby is around six weeks old, as in some women the diabetes doesn't go away. It also means that you have a much higher chance of getting diabetes in later life, so you should try to stick to the healthy living regimen you learnt in pregnancy, and make sure your GP checks your blood sugar every couple of years.

The RCOG has published an excellent patient information leaflet on GDM. Go to www.rcog.org.uk and look under the heading 'patients'.

EXERCISE

We have already outlined the advantages of eating well in pregnancy, and it's also important to know that even a moderate amount of exercise will do both you and your baby good.

Exercise during your pregnancy:

- can improve flexibility, which may help during labour and birth.
- will boost your general fitness and health, which will help you cope with the demands of a new baby.
- will build muscle tone, which may help you regain your pre-pregnancy figure. Core muscle strength will also help you retain your posture and balance during pregnancy.
- can help you sleep.
- can improve circulation.
- can alleviate constipation.
- boosts your immune system.
- will help keep your weight under control if you are finding it hard to resist those cream buns!

Studies have shown that you may have a shorter labour time and fewer delivery complications if you keep fit during pregnancy.

Relaxin, the hormone that relaxes your ligaments and joints in preparation for birth, also makes them more prone to damage, which is why the biggest risk when exercising in pregnancy is injury. You should be aware that if you get excessively hot in the first trimester there is a small possibility that you could damage your baby's nervous system. If you did a particularly vigorous workout before you discovered you were pregnant, don't worry too much: you'd have to have worked yourself into a sweaty frenzy to get hot enough to do any damage.

What kind of exercise should I do?

You may be a committed gym bunny, or perhaps a committed couch potato. Whatever your level of fitness, remember that exercise is to be enjoyed rather than endured in pregnancy.

If you have never exercised regularly before, this is not the time to embark on a rigorous fitness regime, but there are several gentle options that will increase your fitness without you feeling the strain. If you want to join a class, make sure you join an antenatal fitness class: not only is it a great way to meet other pregnant women but you'll also be sure that the exercises are suitable in pregnancy. The NCT runs a Yoga for Pregnancy course that combines a normal antenatal class with yoga. If you need help finding a suitably qualified practitioner in your area, check out the website of the Guild of Pregnancy and Postnatal Exercise Instructors: www.postnatalexercise.co.uk. There are heaps of pregnancy-specific DVDs out there for you to follow at home, but check with your doctor or midwife first if you are in any doubt about exercising.

If you are very fit and exercise regularly, you can continue to do so until your body tells you to slow down. It's OK for you to try to maintain your level of fitness, but don't try to improve it – even the mighty marathon runner Paula Radcliffe had to reduce her training when pregnant.

You may have to accept that you are not going to be at your peak of physical fitness and find new, gentler ways to exercise, but remember this is only temporary and your body will thank you for not overdoing it while it is trying to grow a new life.

Walking

This is the easiest and cheapest exercise option, as you don't have to pay to do it. Try to incorporate a half hour walk into your daily regime. If you have to drive to work, make sure that you take a walk at lunchtime. If you normally take public transport, consider getting off at an earlier stop to walk the last bit of the way or walk all the way if you can. You might find walking in the mornings easier (after the first trimester when you have got past all that sicky stuff) because the growing baby can take his toll on your energy levels.

Swimming

Swimming is ideal pregnancy exercise as the buoyancy of the water will support you and your bump; if you are not very fit you can take it at a gentle pace, or pound up and down the training lanes if you want to up the pace somewhat. The leg action used in the breaststroke can put strain on your lower back and pelvis – particularly if you swim with your head out of the water – so switch to front crawl if you suffer pain in that area.

Cycling

Cycling can be a nice gentle way of getting exercise, particularly in the early months. You should always wear a helmet for safety reasons, and the moment you start feeling unbalanced because of your bump or feel vulnerable cycling in traffic – which can be stressful even when you're not pregnant – switch to brisk walking.

Pilates

Pilates is a low-impact form of exercise and is considered one of the best forms of exercise for a pregnant woman. Pilates helps maintain and improve the condition of both your abdominal and pelvic floor muscles, meaning it can be most beneficial in pregnancy and birth. It also helps you with your posture, which can be a problem when you are waddling around with a big bump. You can buy Pilates in pregnancy DVDs to follow at home if there are no specific classes in your area. If you already do Pilates, tell your instructor you are pregnant, as some exercises may not be suitable for you.

Yoga

Yoga is a great stress buster in pregnancy as the breathing techniques can reduce muscle tension, help you sleep better and generally make you feel more relaxed. Yoga also keeps you supple, which is very helpful when it comes to giving birth as you may have to try a variety of positions to deliver comfortably. It is recommended that you seek medical advice from your doctor or midwife if you have not done yoga before, as there might be physical issues that may prevent you from practising safely. If you already take yoga classes, make sure that your teacher knows you are pregnant, as some yoga positions are not safe in the first trimester and you may need to switch to antenatal-specific yoga.

Aerobic and high-impact exercise

Aerobic (otherwise known as cardiovascular or cardio for short) exercise is exercise that raises your heart rate, and includes power walking, running, dancing and low-impact aerobic classes. These can be safely continued in pregnancy as long as you don't overdo it. If you have never done aerobic exercise before, or you used to but your body is not up to it at the moment, stick to walking briskly or swimming to give your heart and muscles a gentle work out. Pregnancy is not a time to set a new personal best either!

A good tip to check that you are not over-exerting yourself is to do the 'talk test': if you are able to continue a conversation while exercising without catching your breath your body is coping with the activity.

You need to be careful with high-impact exercise, even if you are super fit, because pregnancy makes you more vulnerable to sprains and injuries.

Team sports

If you participate in team sports you really have to judge when to give up; once you have a baby growing inside you, a protective instinct inevitably takes over and most women don't want to indulge in a sport that could harm their baby. As a rule of thumb, once you begin to show, it's probably time to hang up your hockey boots. Sports such as rowing, weight training and tennis will expose you to the risk of muscle and back injuries; anything that involves balance (not easy when you have a huge bump) and the risk of falling, such as gymnastics, horse riding or skiing, is not recommended; and you probably don't need us to tell you that any sport that results in you getting walloped or tackled, like judo, rugby or football, isn't a great idea. Some team sports have rules or restrictions in place for pregnant players so it is worth checking this with your local league.

Exercise dos and don'ts in pregnancy

- **Do** warm up and warm down before and after exercise to minimise the risk of injury.
- **Do** invest in a decent pair of trainers: they will support your feet properly and assist your posture.
- **Do** aim to do half an hour of gentle exercise a day.
- **Do** wear loose, comfy clothes when you are exercising and invest in a sports bra.
- **Do** drink lots of fluids, particularly if you are sweating.
- **Do** listen to your body: if it is tired or achy give exercise a rest or do something gentle rather than strenuous.
- **Don't** exercise strenuously in hot weather.
- **Don't** exercise flat on your back after 16 weeks, as your baby presses on your blood vessels and may make you feel faint.
- **Don't** exercise to lose weight: the aim is to get fit, not thin.

When to stop

If you experience any of the following symptoms while exercising you should stop immediately and seek prompt medical advice:

- dizziness or feeling faint
- headache
- shortness of breath on exertion
- difficulty breathing
- pain or palpitations in your chest
- pain in your abdomen, back, pelvic or pubic area
- weakness in your muscles
- pain or swelling in your leg(s)
- painful uterine contractions
- fewer movements from your baby
- leakage of your amniotic fluid
- vaginal bleeding.

Pelvic floor exercises

If you do no other form of exercise during your pregnancy you really should do your pelvic floor exercises (also called Kegels), and here's why: your pelvic floor is a layer of muscles that form a supportive 'hammock' for your bladder, bowel and uterus. Inevitably it really takes the strain of supporting your baby for nine months and also plays a key role in helping the baby down the birth canal, so it's really important (see www.nhs.uk for more details).

If these muscles become really slack, you will leak urine when you cough, exercise or laugh, so it's important you learn how to do your pelvic floor exercises. The thought of being a slave to panty liners should act as a big enough incentive, but if you want another reason to get squeezing, strong pelvic floor muscles also increase sensitivity during sex and strengthen orgasms, although that might be the last thing on your mind at the moment …

Your pelvic floor muscles are those that stop you peeing mid-flow. (Don't try it when you are actually passing urine: it's damn near impossible when you are pregnant and you should be emptying your bladder every time you pee.)

To do your pelvic floor exercises:
- tighten those muscles you would use when peeing and pooing
- don't be tempted to tighten your tummy, buttock or thigh muscles as these won't help the pelvic floor
- once you have identified the correct muscles, try squeezing and releasing them quickly 10 times
- next, squeeze slowly and try to hold the muscles tightly for up to 10 seconds before relaxing: repeat this 10 times
- try both sets of squeezes between four and six times a day.

A tip is to put random coloured stickers around the house, in your handbag, or in the car. You don't have to tell anyone what they are for and they'll act as a reminder to do a few squeezes. The beauty of these exercises is that no one will know you are doing them!

'HAZARDOUS' ACTIVITIES

Being pregnant can mean that you have to change your lifestyle: not only in terms of what you eat and drink, but also how you carry out your beauty routine or clean your home. Here are a few areas that you'll need to review now that you're pregnant.

Meeting other people

Small ones …

Your friends' children may pose a hazard when you are pregnant because toddlers are prone to contagious diseases such as chickenpox and Parvovirus

B19 (slapped cheek disease). As most of us have had these childhood illnesses you should be immune anyway, but if you didn't contract them as a child and you do come into contact with someone contagious, contact your GP or midwife (but don't go into the maternity unit) so they can run tests and treat you and your baby if necessary. Of people brought up in the UK, 90% have had chickenpox, but if you haven't yet, then you could discuss having a vaccination with your GP – this is not available on the NHS.

And big ones …

Bird flu and swine flu (H1N1), not to mention the old-fashioned regular influenza, are all things that you might pick up from the people around you. Pregnant women are more prone to developing severe or dangerous complications from flu, so the advice is to have the vaccination if you are pregnant in autumn or winter. You can't wrap yourself in cotton wool and avoid human contact for nine months, but you are more likely to catch a contagious disease because your immune system is weaker than normal. If you do get unwell make sure you seek medical advice quickly, and ensure you maintain really good hand hygiene, washing hands before and after food preparation, and before and after going to the toilet. Group A streptococcus causes a sore throat and a cold, but if it gets into the uterus via the vagina it can make you or the baby very unwell.

Following a whooping cough outbreak in 2012, pregnant women are advised to have a booster vaccination after 16 weeks; this was recently revised from 28 weeks. This is to ensure the baby is born with enough protection to last until his own vaccines are due (when he is two months old).

 Words from the professionals

As testing in pregnancy for Rubella immunity is no longer routine, check your vaccination record and if you have not had the MMR vaccine, discuss this with your GP (if possible before you are pregnant, as MMR vaccines cannot be given in pregnancy).

To tan or not to tan?

Some pregnant women suffer from uneven skin pigmentation during pregnancy (chloasma), and exposure to the sun or UV rays can make it worse. If you do start getting uneven brown patches on your skin, remember to wear a hat and slap on the sunscreen when you are out in the sun.

Using sunbeds in pregnancy is not recommended: firstly because research has linked increased UV rays to folic acid deficiency, and secondly because you increase the risk of chloasma. Avoid tanning pills and injections altogether while pregnant as most brands are unlicensed and untested.

If you can't live without fake tan, be aware that your skin is much more sensitive when you are pregnant, so do a patch test first to check that you don't get an allergic reaction. Some experts recommend you don't use fake tan, presumably because of the chemical content (you only have to smell the stuff to know it's laden with them), so it's down to you whether you can bear to be 'pale and interesting' instead.

Hot tubs et al

Give saunas, jacuzzis, steam baths and hot tubs a miss during pregnancy. We have already explained that overheating, particularly in the first trimester, can affect your baby's nervous system, which is why anything that raises your body temperature such as hot tubs and saunas should be avoided when you are pregnant. Later in pregnancy, excessive heat can push up your baby's heart rate and lower your blood pressure – making you feel dizzy or faint – so that's another two good reasons why you should give them a miss.

Likewise, although there's nothing nicer than lying in the bath having a long soak when you are pregnant, given the reasons above, do make sure it's not too hot. If the water temperature turns your skin pink, turn on the cold tap!

Aromatherapy

Aromatherapy has been shown to be very effective in alleviating certain pregnancy ailments, but some essential oils can be risky when treating pregnant women, so it is important that you see a qualified practitioner who is registered with the Aromatherapy Council.

Hair dye

Experts cannot say for *certain* that chemicals in hair dye are completely safe for use in pregnancy, which is why some recommend that you avoid colouring your hair in the first trimester, when your baby's brain and nervous system are developing at the most dramatic rate. There are no studies that say with absolute certainty that it does your baby any harm, though; so if maintaining your hair colour is fundamental to who you are as a person, then carry on and don't lose any sleep over it, because modern hair dyes are probably safer than they have ever been.

If you do like to give your hair colour a boost and are worried about using chemicals on your scalp, you can always use a semi-permanent rinse which isn't as strong, henna-based dyes, or consider highlights or lowlights to give your lacklustre locks a lift.

Do remember that your hormones may affect your hair's condition so you might get a different colour or texture than expected, and you may also suffer an unexpected allergic reaction, so do a patch test first.

At home

Gardening

Wear gloves and wash your hands thoroughly after gardening, as soil can contain the toxoplasmosis bug. There's no reason why you shouldn't garden throughout your pregnancy, as it is good exercise, but make sure you protect your back and leave any heavy digging to someone else.

Painting

Modern water-based paints such as emulsions should be completely safe for you to use, as they are very unlikely to have a harmful effect on your baby. As there has not been extensive recent research on this type of paint, though, the NHS recommends you avoid painting in the first trimester as a precaution.

We do know that solvent-based paints, varnishes and brush cleaners are likely to cause more harm than water-based ones due to their chemical content, so it's recommended you don't use these during pregnancy if possible.

If you are renovating a property or room in preparation for your baby, make sure that you don't strip any paint off yourself. Paint dating from before 1978 contains lead, which could be harmful to your unborn child, so leave that job to the professionals or your partner.

There are lots of eco-friendly organic paints on the market that contain no nasty chemicals, so consider these for your baby's nursery if you're worried.

Electrical appliances

There hasn't been extensive study in this area but the received wisdom is that modern microwaves are safe. If your microwave is very old or doesn't work well, it might be prudent to invest in a new one.

Electric blankets should be used with caution. It is dangerous to overheat your body during pregnancy, so if you use one keep the temperature low so the bed is warm but not hot. Some people worry about the electromagnetic field arising from the electricity used to heat the blanket being dangerous for their baby, but there is no definitive evidence to prove this. If it worries you and you can't live without a bit of extra heat in bed, why not switch to a trusty hot water bottle?

Household chemicals and cleaning products

There isn't firm evidence on the dangers of exposure to household chemicals, but to be on the safe side it's wise to avoid powerful products such as pesticides and oven cleaners.

If you are cleaning it also makes sense to protect your hands with gloves and ventilate the room by opening a window. Most items you use daily – such as anti-bacterial spray in the kitchen and bathroom – should be fine, but try not to inhale them.

If you are anxious about chemicals you can always make your own natural cleaning products. Baking soda is an efficient powdered cleanser for greasy areas like pots, sinks and ovens; a solution of vinegar and water is perfect for window cleaning and mopping down surfaces in the kitchen.

Household pets

It's recommended that you wash your hands after any contact with pets because animal waste does tend to harbour bacteria. In our experience this isn't always convenient – as anyone who has ever owned a cat or dog would know – but it does make sense to wash your hands regularly if you have animals in the house, particularly before eating.

Computers

If you use a computer at home and at work (there's more about specific risks at work in the next chapter), you'll be relieved to know that there is no evidence of any risks associated with their regular use.

Out and about

Holidays
Flying

Flying is generally considered safe in pregnancy, although some airlines refuse to let you fly after 28 weeks, while others insist you have a doctor's note certifying you are fit to travel. Policies vary from airline to airline, so it is important you know your dates before you make a booking. If you have diabetes or placenta praevia, or have had issues with blood pressure or bleeding in your pregnancy, it would be sensible to check with your doctor before you fly. There is an increased risk of DVT (deep vein thrombosis – see page 65) when you are pregnant and flying can increase the risk further, so ensure you move about as much as possible, rotate your ankles while you are sitting down, and invest in a pair of flight socks (long, over-the-knee support socks). You can get these from Boots or at the airport and, while they may not be glamorous, they can be a lifesaver (literally). If you are at risk of pre-term delivery, take extra care when planning a trip to make sure you don't deliver away from family and friends.

Insurance and medical treatment abroad

You need to take out adequate travel insurance and make sure you know what you are covered for before you go anywhere, in case you need local treatment at a surgery or hospital. Read the small print because some insurers won't cover care for you in pregnancy or your baby, or repatriate either of you if you go into early labour. If you are travelling in Europe, make sure you travel with your European Health Insurance Card (you can apply online at www.ehic.org. uk), as it currently entitles you to basic medical care in other EU countries (except in Switzerland) – but beware regulations may change following the

Brexit negotiations. Make sure you take a photocopy of your pregnancy medical notes and your GP's number with you.

If you are going to an area where mosquitoes are a problem, think very carefully about whether the trip is essential. Take an insect sleeping net and use an insect repellent containing DEET, which is safe for use during pregnancy and breastfeeding. It's not advisable to go to a country where malaria is prevalent as this disease can be harmful to you and your baby. If you really have to go, speak to your doctor about anti-malarial drugs that are suitable to take in pregnancy. It is better to take the tablets than risk getting malaria.

If you are planning a babymoon, or are having an exotic holiday or honeymoon during pregnancy, remember that some countries require vaccinations that are unsafe in pregnancy. Your GP can advise you, or you can check out the MASTA (Medical Advisory Services for Travellers Abroad) website for more information: www.masta-travel-health.com.

 Words from the professionals

Zika infection remains a risk in many South and Central American, Caribbean, African and Asian countries. Check the latest advice on www.gov.uk before travelling. There is concern that the Zika virus can cross the placenta and cause a potentially serious problem in your baby's brain: microcephaly.

Foreign travel dos and don'ts

- **Do** check with your doctor about what medical items are safe to take with you, like oral rehydration in case of diarrhoea, antihistamines in case of bites, etc. It will be much easier to take a mini medical kit with you than to try to explain you are pregnant and in need of 'x' in a foreign pharmacy.

- **Do** stay out of the sun between 11am and 3pm, and always wear a sunhat and sun protection to stop you overheating.

- **Do** drink lots of bottled water to keep yourself hydrated, and clean your teeth with it if you are concerned about the quality of the tap water.

- **Do** be careful around wet pool areas to avoid a fall.

- **Do** travel with a mini hand sanitiser in your bag to freshen up your hands, cutlery, etc.

- **Don't** eat anything you think has been hanging around or is not properly cooked.

Theme parks

You might have to curb your love of thrills and spills when you are pregnant, as many rides have rapid stops and starts which could damage the uterus. Water slides should also be approached with caution. Most theme park rides and pools display clear signage stipulating their suitability for pregnant women, and our advice would be to stick to the rules; let's face it, becoming a parent is usually the mother of all rollercoaster rides.

Extreme sports

Thrill seekers who enjoy extreme sports such as hang-gliding, rock climbing, bungee jumping or skydiving will have to give these activities a miss for a while, and there's probably not a doctor in the land who would disagree with us.

High-altitude sports

High-altitude sports such as mountaineering and hot air ballooning are officially discouraged, because a change in altitude levels means exposure to lower oxygen levels and this can be harmful for the baby.

Scuba diving

Scuba diving is also a no-no in pregnancy because there is evidence that your baby could be put at risk of decompression sickness (aka the bends) and it can also increase the likelihood of miscarriage.

Down on the farm

Pregnant women are advised to avoid sheep during lambing periods, according to the latest guidelines from the Department of Health, as there is a risk of catching chlamydophila abortus, toxoplasmosis and listeriosis from aborted sheep, newborn lambs or their afterbirth. If you do go to a farm or farm park, your best bet is to avoid sheep altogether if possible. If this is impossible, make sure you don't touch, feed or milk the lambs or ewes, avoid contact with their bedding or straw, and wash your hands scrupulously after leaving.

Having said all that ...

The list of dos and don'ts can be pretty daunting and cause a lot of unnecessary worry for some pregnant ladies. Try to enjoy your pregnancy: have fun, relax and listen to your body. If you are worried about doing something, don't do it. If you feel you have bags of energy, feel free to be a social butterfly! Just remember to take it easy and try to get some rest. Take life a bit slower!

5

My career

There is no doubt that having a baby is going to have an impact on your career to some degree, but how pregnancy and birth affect your working life will depend on your type of job and personal circumstances. In this chapter we take you through the common legal, physical and emotional issues regarding work and pregnancy, and explain how best to deal with them.

YOUR RIGHTS AND RESPONSIBILITIES

It may not be quite as exciting as thinking about names or nursery decor, but it is vitally important that you are up to speed on the latest government legislation regarding pregnancy and maternity leave.

The main government website is a good place to start (www.gov.uk). In the Working, jobs and pensions section there is a fairly comprehensive Maternity category that gives up-to-date information on your legal rights, so make sure you check it out, as it is possible that things have changed since this book was written.

If you work for a large corporation it is probable that it will be totally au fait with any new rules, but if you work for a small company it might not be so on the ball with any changes in the law. What follows is a basic guide to your legal rights as a pregnant employee, although entitlements do vary depending on a wealth of factors, including length of service, type of contract, employer, so you'll need to do your homework to find out exactly what you're entitled to.

When should I tell?

Legally, you have to tell your boss by the time you are 25 weeks pregnant, but the chances are that everyone will have noticed if you leave it that late!

Many women like to keep mum about the news until they have had their first scan, but if you are really suffering with morning sickness and running to the bathroom every five minutes, you might want to share your news with a supportive boss or trusted work colleague so that you can have some moral or physical support. If you work in a female-dominated environment it's quite likely that one of the other women will notice that you are permanently green or camping out in the loo, and you might find your 'secret' more difficult to keep than you first imagined.

Your employer has a legal requirement to keep you safe during your pregnancy and should do a risk assessment to check that you can still carry out your working duties safely while you are pregnant (see page 123). Therefore, the earlier you let them know, the safer your baby will be.

If you work in a small company your pregnancy leave might have a significant impact on the business, so if you can give your employer plenty of notice it will give them the opportunity to make plans to cover your absence.

What do I need to do and say?

You should put in writing when your baby is due and when you would like your maternity leave and maternity pay to start. If you change your mind and decide you want to carry on working until nearer your due date you should give your employer 28 days' notice, but many bosses will give you some flexibility on this issue, as it may be in their interest to keep you at work as long as possible.

You also need to show your employer a copy of your Maternity Certificate (MATB1) that you get from your midwife after 21 weeks and that confirms your due date.

What will happen then?

Your employer must assume that you are going to take your full entitlement of 52 weeks' maternity leave (unless you tell them that you are planning to return without taking the full amount of leave).

Your employer must write to you within 28 days of receiving notification of your pregnancy dates, confirming the date you are due to return to work.

If you already know that you can't afford to take your full 52 weeks of maternity leave, you *can* tell your boss at this early stage that you will be returning early. If your circumstances change and you change your mind once the baby is born, as long as you give eight weeks' notice you can still take the full entitlement, even if you said you would be returning earlier. If you don't know whether you will be off for the whole time or not, it is best to hedge your bets and assume you will take your full entitlement: you can always change your mind as long as you give the two months' notice.

EMPLOYERS' RIGHTS AND RESPONSIBILITIES

As soon as you tell your employer that you are pregnant, they must:

- carry out a risk assessment to identify any risk to you or your child's health

- allow you paid time off to attend antenatal appointments

- ensure you are not treated unfairly by your manager or other colleagues

- plan for your leave – you can take up to 52 weeks' leave (you must not return to work for the first two weeks after the birth of your baby, or the first four weeks if you work in a factory).

Within 28 days of receiving your maternity leave dates, your employer must write to you telling you when you are due back at work and how you will be paid Statutory Maternity Pay (SMP), or, if you do not qualify for SMP, send you Form SMP1 which you will need to complete to apply for maternity allowance. If you work part time, your entitlements to leave and maternity pay are pro rata.

During maternity leave:

- you and your employer can make reasonable contact with each other. Your employer should agree with you the kind of contact you will have during your leave, for example, how your employer will let you know about any changes happening at work, including job vacancies, and whether there will be opportunities for you to attend training or other events.

- you can work for up to 10 days. These are known as KIT (Keeping In Touch) days (see page 132).

- if your employer makes contributions to an occupational pension, they must continue to make these for the whole time you are receiving SMP or contractual maternity pay.

Before you return to work:

- you must give your employer eight weeks' notice if you change your mind about the date you return to work. If you do not do this, and your employer needs more notice than you have given, they can postpone your return until the required eight weeks' notice has passed (although they cannot postpone your return to work beyond the 52-week leave period).

- if you make a request for flexible working, including part-time work, your employer must seriously consider the request. Your employer can turn down this request on genuine business grounds or agree to a different arrangement with you.

- if you tell your employer that you will be breastfeeding, they must talk to you about any arrangements they will need to make to enable you to do this, as well as complete a risk assessment and remove any risk they find.

WORKING OUT YOUR FINANCES

Sadly, for many of us, the issue about returning to work is governed by finance rather than emotion. Many women would love to stay at home or work part time, but their financial situation dictates that they continue their career to pay the mortgage and the bills. Some women can't take their full maternity leave because they simply can't afford to manage on SMP.

Before your baby is born it's really valuable to do the sums to see if you can survive the full 52 weeks' leave, and useful to work out if you could manage on a reduced salary if you did cut your hours or days after returning to work.

You also need to factor in childcare costs because you will probably have to pay someone to look after your child, unless you have a willing parent or relative close by who is prepared to care for your baby for free.

Many couples spend pregnancy squirrelling as much cash away as they can; this is good practice because you will incur numerous baby-related costs after your baby is born.

Take a long, hard look at your finances before you start considering your maternity leave options to make sure you make the best decision possible.

MATERNITY LEAVE

If you are an employee you will be entitled to the maximum amount of leave set by the government, called statutory maternity leave (SML). This period is 52 weeks and is made up of 26 weeks of ordinary maternity leave (OML) and 26 weeks of additional maternity leave (AML). This means you are entitled to a full year off work if you are an employee. Your length of service, rate of pay or hours of work do not affect your statutory maternity leave.

You do not have to take all your statutory maternity leave, but legally you have to take two 'compulsory' weeks off after the baby is born or four weeks off if you work in a factory.

If you are a casual or agency worker or you are self-employed, different rules apply, so you need to check out your legal employment status to see what you are entitled to. Visit www.dwp.gov.uk for more information on this.

You can begin OML up to 11 weeks before your baby is due, although most people prefer to wait so that they can afford to spend more time off after their baby is born. You can be creative with your annual leave, though, and use some of this before your maternity leave starts to make your maternity leave last longer. You are also entitled to your allocated annual leave allowance while you are on maternity leave, which you could use at the end of your maternity leave.

Your basic rights

There are a number of rights that pregnant women are entitled to by law. These are known as statutory rights and are:

- the right to take time off for antenatal care
- the right to work in a safe environment
- the right to claim discrimination and unfair dismissal if dismissed because of pregnancy and maternity leave
- the right to take up to 52 weeks' maternity leave
- the right of some pregnant women to statutory maternity pay (SMP)
- the right to return to work after having the baby.

MATERNITY PAY

Statutory Maternity Pay (SMP)

Your work may have its own maternity pay scheme which you may qualify for. If not, you may qualify for SMP, paid by the government. If you do not qualify for SMP your employer must give you Form SMP1. You may be eligible for Maternity Allowance instead (see page 121).

To qualify for SMP you must have been:

- employed by the same employers for a continuous period of at least 26 weeks into the 15th week before the week your baby is due (the qualifying week)

- earning, on average, an amount that at least equals the lower earnings limit which applies on the Saturday at the end of your qualifying week. (The 2019 lower earnings limit was £118 a week. This is the amount you have to earn before you pay National Insurance contributions.)

To make a claim for SMP you must:

- tell your employer when you want your SMP to start

- provide medical evidence of the date your baby is due.

SMP is paid for 39 weeks, and is split:

- at 90% of your average gross weekly earnings, with no upper limit, for the first six weeks

- at either the standard rate of £148.68 (2019 figure), or 90% of your average gross weekly earnings, for the remaining 33 weeks – whichever is lower.

Your employer will usually pay you in the same way and at the same time as your normal wages.

You must use the date your baby is due to work out your SMP for that pregnancy.

Returning to work while receiving SMP

You can work for up to 10 days during your maternity pay period (MPP) for the employer paying your SMP without this affecting your SMP entitlement. These are called Keeping In Touch (KIT) days (see page 132). If you then do any further work for your employer during your MPP, you will lose SMP for each week in your MPP that you do that work.

If you start work for a new employer after your baby is born (an employer who did not employ you in the 15th week before your baby was due), you must tell the employer paying your SMP and your SMP must stop.

Key facts about SMP

- Go onto www.gov.uk and uae the interactive tool to help you work out what your SMP will be.

- If you decide not to return to work after receiving your SMP, you do not have to pay anything back to your employer.

- If you take time off work because of pregnancy-related medical issues from four weeks before your due date, your employer is legally entitled to start paying you SMP and to assume you have commenced your OML, even if you had planned to work up until 38 weeks.

- If you work for two employers you may be entitled to receive SMP from both.

- If you start employment with a new company while you are still pregnant your SMP is not affected, but if you start with a new company after the baby is born you must tell your previous employer, who will then stop paying you your SMP.

- If you are ill after the birth, you may be able to claim statutory sick pay after your SMP payments finish.

- If a baby is stillborn after 24 weeks, or is born after that date and doesn't survive, his mother is still entitled to SMP.

Your company's maternity scheme

Some companies will offer additional maternity pay, paid on top of SMP. Ask if you are entitled to this (most stipulate a minimum service requirement), and check the details – if you decide not to return to work, you may have to pay back some or all the money paid in excess of SMP. Some generous companies let you keep the money, regardless of whether you return to work.

Maternity Allowance

If you aren't entitled to SMP, you'll be entitled to Maternity Allowance if:

- you have worked for 26 weeks in the last 66 weeks (this could be in lots of different chunks or for different employers: it can also include self-employed work)

- you earned more than £30 for 13 of those weeks (you can choose the weeks when you've earned the most, combine wages from different jobs, and it can include overtime, bonuses, or sick pay).

You'll receive £148.68 per week (or 90% of your earnings, whichever is less) or £27 a week for 14 or 39 weeks. It will depend on your eligibility – use the maternity entitlement calculator on www.gov.uk to work it out.

I'm self-employed – what do I get?

If you are self-employed, you are not entitled to SMP, but you will be entitled to Maternity Allowance if:

- you have worked for 26 weeks in the last 66 weeks (either for yourself or for an employer)

- you have 13 weeks where you have paid Class 2 NI (National Insurance) contributions or held a certificate of small earnings exemption.

If you have got 13 weeks of Class 2 NI contributions, you are entitled to the full amount of £148.68. If you have the certificate, you will be entitled to £27 a week. If you own a limited company and pay yourself through PAYE, you will qualify for SMP if you meet the conditions.

Sure Start Maternity Grant

This is a one-off non-repayable grant of £500 to go towards the cost of raising your child. This grant is available only to first-time mums-to-be on a low income or in receipt of certain benefits. Go to www.gov.uk for more details. If you live in Scotland you cannot get this grant, but you may apply for a Pregnancy and Baby payment instead.

Unpaid parental leave

Unpaid parental leave is available to each parent for each child. You are allowed to take 18 weeks' leave for each child, up to their 18th birthday. The leave must be taken in blocks of one week, with not more than four weeks being taken each year. It is intended to be used, for example, to look at new schools, or settle children into childcare arrangements. See more details of this, and how it can be used, at www.gov.uk/parental-leave, or ask your HR department if you wish to take some. The parental leave is always in addition to any maternity or paternity leave taken.

WHAT ABOUT PARTNERS?

Eligible parents (same-sex parents included) can now take leave at different times or double up by taking leave at the same time, for up to 50 weeks, 37 of which will be paid. Mothers must still take the first two weeks after the birth of their child, but can then exchange traditional maternity leave for Shared Parental Leave (SPL). Both parents have a flexible choice of how to split up their 50 weeks of leave – ie whether to take it in one continuous block or in smaller chunks of time. For example, the mother could decide to take off 10 weeks after the birth, and then she and her partner would be able to choose how to split the remaining 40 weeks of leave. She could choose to take another 30 weeks and her partner take 10, or they could both take 20 weeks at different or at coinciding times.

The difference from the old rules is that the leave does not have to be taken all in one go, even if only the mother chooses to take up SPL as opposed to traditional maternity leave. A parent can book up to three blocks of leave during the child's first year, and have to give their employer eight weeks' notice of each block. A mother can also let her employer know before her baby is born that she doesn't plan to use all of her 52 weeks' maternity leave and wants to convert some of it into SPL. Her partner could then use this leave in the first few weeks after birth, so both parents are on leave at the same time.

To take shared leave, one parent must have been an employee with at least 26 weeks of service with the same employer by the end of the 15th week before the baby is due, or when matched with an adopted child. The other parent must have worked for at least 26 weeks in the 66 weeks leading up to the due date and have earned at least £30 a week in 13 of the 66 weeks. Self-employed parents, and a parent not in work at the time of the birth, can still qualify.

SPL pay is £148.68 a week, or 90% of an employee's average weekly earnings, whichever is lower. This is the same as statutory maternity pay, except that during the first six weeks statutory maternity pay amounts to 90% of whatever the employee earns, with no maximum. Some employers may offer an enhanced package but there is no legal requirement for them to do so.

SPL pay is only given for 37 weeks. The remaining 13 weeks of leave entitlement, if taken, is unpaid. Go to www.gov.uk for more information.

Stay-at-home partners

All evidence suggests that the uptake of SPL since its introduction in 2015 has been low, with the government predicting that initially a maximum of 8% of partners will likely take the opportunity to be at home with their children. This is not necessarily suggestive of the scheme's failure, though. Societal change takes time: this low figure reflects the uptake when Sweden introduced the same scheme, 40 years ago, and now it is at nearly 90%. All the evidence suggests there's a changing tide, and the last 10 years have seen a dramatic increase in the number of stay-at-home dads.

YOUR MATERNITY RIGHTS AT WORK

Antenatal care

You are legally allowed to have paid time off to attend antenatal appointments. This includes parentcraft classes and hospital tours as well as your routine appointments, but you may need to show your boss or employer evidence that you have a hospital visit and you are not just bunking off on a shopping trip.

Your partner does not have the legal right to have paid time off to attend antenatal appointments with you, but if his employer is 'family friendly' they might let him take the time off and make it up at a later date.

Health and safety at work during pregnancy

You need to take care of yourself at work when you are pregnant, and that doesn't just mean legally and financially. You need to ensure that you have adequate health and safety protection as well.

Once you have formally notified your employer of your pregnancy in writing, they must carry out a specific risk assessment based on your needs as an employee. By law your employer has to protect your health and safety during pregnancy, and failure to do so is classed as sex discrimination.

If any risks are identified, your employer must inform you and tell you how they will ensure you are not exposed to them.

Potential workplace risks include:

- lifting or carrying heavy loads

- standing or sitting for long periods of time

- exposure to any of the following: infectious diseases; lead; hazardous chemicals; radioactive material; excessive noise; extremes of temperature, shock, or vibration

- work-related stress

- workstation set-up: seating and posture

- long working hours

- mental or physical fatigue

- threat of violence.

If there is a risk to you or your baby and your employer cannot adjust your conditions or hours to protect you from it, legally they have to find you suitable alternative work on the same pay and conditions. If they cannot meet this request you can be suspended on full pay until they can.

Don't be nervous about raising the issue of health and safety while you're pregnant. You might feel like you're being pushy or making a fuss, but it is your legal right to be protected by your employer, so make sure you are being properly cared for. Your safety and the safety of your baby are paramount. You might find that you are a company's first pregnant employee or that there is already a thorough health and safety policy in place. Whatever your circumstances, make sure you keep pushing it until you are happy.

Being able to work

You should also be aware that if you have medical issues arising from your pregnancy that affect your ability to do your present job, you need to make sure that you get a note from your GP or midwife explaining the problem. This ensures your employer can eliminate certain duties from your workload or accommodate you in a different role within the organisation if necessary.

Applying for a new job when you are pregnant

If you apply for a position in a new company during pregnancy, it counts as sex discrimination for them not to give you the job because you are pregnant (although proving that may be quite difficult in a court of law). Obviously, if it is early days and you are not showing, any prospective employer will judge you in the same way as any other candidate, and if they give you the job and you subsequently tell them you are pregnant they cannot change their minds and retract the job offer.

Applying for a promotion

Many women worry that once they are pregnant any chance of a promotion flies out of the window. However, your employers have a legal obligation to make you aware of any promotions coming up and invite you to apply for them. We'd love to say that your pregnancy should have no bearing on whether you get the job, but sadly this is not always the case. At least you have the legal right to be considered for any promotion, and if a candidate with less experience is offered the job over you, you may well have a case to show that your employer is guilty of sex discrimination.

When you are the boss

Responsibility to your employees

The people who work for you may be worried about what happens to the business in your absence, so make sure you have a rough contingency plan in place before you announce the news to your staff to allay their fears.

Responsibility to yourself

You have to do your own risk assessments and ensure that you are keeping yourself safe and protected at work. For the sake of your baby and your fellow employees, make sure you don't overdo it: if your body tells you to slow down or stop you should do so; that's what you would expect the people working for you to do and you should be no different.

Responsibility for your future and that of your company

You need to sit down and work out how long you can afford to take off in the personal and financial sense, and also work out how long your company can survive without you while you take maternity leave. You shouldn't rush back to work before you're ready, but you will need to make sure you have an excellent plan in place for how the company will be run while you are away.

A COMFORTABLE WORKING PREGNANCY

Even if you don't have any specific risks involved with your job, everyday working conditions can take their toll on even the healthiest pregnant women. It's useful to think about your working day and see how you might have to adapt it now you're pregnant to make you and your baby as comfortable as possible.

A working pregnancy can be enjoyable and not merely endurable. Here are some tips on how to make working while you're pregnant as comfortable as possible.

Commuting

Driving

There are benefits to driving to work: you can open the windows easily if you need air; you can stop if you are going to be sick; and you don't have to put up with all the weird and wonderful smells (that you can't bear with your pregnancy-heightened senses) that travelling on public transport inevitably brings. However, one of the hazards of driving while pregnant is that you may be slightly more accident-prone if you are suffering with 'preg head', and you'll need to make sure your bump is protected in case of any knocks.

If you drive to work, make sure your driving position is comfortable, protect your back with a cushion and take a break and stretch your legs if the commute is a long one. It's also a good idea to invest in a pregnancy seat belt. There are a variety of styles on offer, from cushioned straps to contraptions that actually change the position of the seat belt so it doesn't lie directly across your tummy.

Public transport

Obviously the stress of your commute will depend on the distance, mode of transport and how congested the route becomes. There's no doubt that a rural bus journey is likely to be more pleasant (and scenic) than a trip on the London Underground during rush hour, but if you are feeling tired, groggy or sick, both will be equally torturous.

If your commute is getting you down, you can reasonably ask for a change in start or finish times to avoid the worst of the rush hour (even 15 minutes can make a difference), and it may be feasible for you to work from home for part or all of the day.

It's ironic that in the first trimester – when you feel that you need a seat most – you won't get one, because you won't be showing and no one will know you are pregnant. Even when you have a bump the size of a football stuffed inside your jumper, there's no guarantee you will get a seat.

If you feel that you need a seat, just pluck up the courage and ask – most people normally oblige. Or you could wear a 'Baby on Board' badge – available online and at some ticket offices. Keep a bottle of water and a snack in your bag in case of a breakdown or emergency. During pregnancy you have a different centre of gravity, so swap those heels for flats when commuting, to prevent trips, slips or falls.

Sickness

It's pretty rotten feel sick at work. We've given you some tips on how to deal with pregnancy nausea earlier on in the book (see page 68), but sadly there's not a great deal you can do to hide the problem at work, even if you are trying to keep your pregnancy a secret in the early days.

If your sickness is mornings only and you have a sympathetic boss, you could spill the beans and work from home in the mornings, or change your working hours so that you come into the office once the sickness has subsided. It is likely, though, that your co-workers will cotton on to the fact that you are pregnant, and you might not want to tell them until you have had your first scan and know the baby is OK.

If you suffer severe morning sickness you probably won't be able to keep it from your colleagues; indeed, you may have to get yourself signed off to prevent you getting dehydrated. Your employer may not be very sympathetic to your condition if you need to be signed off, but legally there's nothing they can do about it.

If you are suffering, think about flexible working patterns you could do (for example, could you work at home for a couple of days a week or work flexi-time?), figure out if there is any work you could hand to a colleague and go to your boss with a solution. It will be better to present possible solutions rather than just asking to be signed off.

Reduced hours

You have a right to ask for reduced working hours during pregnancy, but legally your employer doesn't have to agree to it if it doesn't suit the needs of the business; if you do cut your workload and your salary goes down it will affect the amount of SMP you receive when you go on maternity leave.

Pregnancy-related illness

If you are ill when you are pregnant you are entitled to have this time off as paid sick leave – unless you are ill in the four weeks before your due date, in which case your employer has a legal right to start your maternity leave and pay you SMP. Any pregnancy-related sickness should be treated the same as normal sick leave, and your employer is guilty of sex discrimination if they threaten you with a disciplinary action or sacking for taking time off for illness in pregnancy. If you do need to take time off for illness or health issues during pregnancy, it is important that you get a note confirming you have a problem from your GP or midwife. Not only will it confirm your absence is legitimate, but it would also be useful if you need evidence at an employment tribunal should your employer start getting nasty about you being off work.

Baby brain

Studies contradict each other as to whether 'baby brain' is real or in the mind; however, there is no doubt that many pregnant women find it difficult to keep the same levels of concentration when they are pregnant, and that can lead to problems at work.

Here are some tips to help you combat your 'baby brain'.

- Write a 'to do' list of jobs every morning when you get into work to make sure that you get all your tasks completed.

- If possible, schedule meetings when you are most alert. If you are liveliest in the morning and doziest after lunch make sure you try to have breakfast or brunch meetings.

- Eat and drink regularly to keep your energy levels up as this will assist concentration.

Stress

The jury is out on whether stress at work has an effect on your baby – a recent study showed that a baby's development might improve as a result of moderate work stress, whereas another showed that a fetus as young as 18 weeks could sense anxiety in the mother. What we do know is that excessive stress can raise your blood pressure (which can cause problems in pregnancy), and can also manifest itself physically in the form of insomnia and headaches, so if you are really feeling the stress at work you should speak to your boss or HR manager about finding a solution. They have a duty to try to alleviate or remove the factors that are causing you grief where possible, or adjust your conditions or hours accordingly.

If things get really bad or if work stress is affecting your wellbeing and that of your child, you can speak to your GP about getting signed off.

Exhaustion

Exhaustion can hit you during any part of your pregnancy: your surging hormones can completely wipe you out in the first trimester, and by the third, the sheer effort of carrying round your baby can make you so tired you just want to weep.

Many pregnant women have trouble sleeping, which exacerbates the problem, and if your job is of a physical nature or involves standing for long periods of time it's bound to make the problem worse.

To help you avoid feeling totally exhausted:

- take a power nap. If you are struggling to get through the day, a short snooze for around 15–20 minutes can really boost your energy levels. Try not to nap for longer, though, as studies have shown you can wake up feeling worse. In theory your employers should provide a place for you to rest, although in reality this might not be practical.

- take regular breaks. Most employees are entitled to breaks during the day, so make sure you take yours. If you have nowhere to escape to, turn your PC off, close your eyes and relax for a few minutes; if you have a rest or leisure area, make the most of it and get away from your working environment to refresh your brain and boost your energy levels.

- If your job involves long periods standing up it makes sense to work in a pair of comfortable shoes; ballerina flats are very fashionable, so you don't have to sacrifice style for comfort (you'll just look shorter!). We covered back problems in pregnancy on page 52. Standing all day can make it worse, so make sure that you sit down at regular intervals to give your body a rest; your boss should provide a chair or stool for you to do this.

Are you sitting comfortably?

If you sit for long periods of time, you increase your risk of developing deep vein thrombosis and are more likely to feel dizzy and faint when you stand up. You may also increase the risk of back or pelvic pain; therefore it is important that you create a comfortable position in which to carry out your working duties.

Here's what you should do to ensure you're sitting correctly.

- Make sure your chair is high enough: your feet should be flat on the floor with your hips slightly higher than your knees. You can raise your feet with a box or stool if necessary.

- Your computer screen should be directly in front of you, with your eyes level with the middle of the screen.

- Support your spine with a cushion placed between your chair and the small of your back.

- Keep your posture erect. Sit up straight with your shoulders relaxed and don't slouch.

- Try to keep your pelvis tilted slightly upwards when sitting.

- Take regular breaks; get up and walk around for a couple of minutes at least twice an hour.

- Don't cross your legs when you sit down: it twists your spine, restricts circulation and may encourage the formation of varicose veins.

- If you are struggling to get out of your chair, ask your boss for one with armrests.

- As your bump increases, adjust your chair height accordingly. If your current work station can't accommodate a growing belly, ask your boss to move you or change your current office set-up.

Dealing with an unsympathetic boss or colleague

In an ideal world everyone would be delighted that you are pregnant, but unfortunately many pregnant women encounter some sort of hostility at work once their pregnancy is announced. You may have the law on your side, but that doesn't prevent people being mean, sarcastic or petty, and you may find that the attitudes of your boss or your colleagues change once you are pregnant.

You may find your commitment being tested, your working hours queried or your colleagues resentful of the time you take off. This can take its toll on you when you are feeling a bit wobbly and emotional, but there are some options open to you.

- Work with your boss to make sure that he or she has plenty of advance notice of absences and appointments; you are entitled to take this time off, but operations will run more smoothly if people can plan for you not being around.

- Try to look at it from your boss's perspective: sometimes they get quite frightened at the prospect of losing a key worker and this can manifest itself in them behaving negatively towards you. If you think there's a really good chance you'll be returning to work, then assure them of your intentions.

- Get someone on your side: sometimes it's helpful to have a work friend battling your corner and supporting you.

- Grin and bear it. You're going to have a whole year off soon with your baby, and this is only a short-term hurdle to your long-term future.

If you do feel that you are being mistreated, make sure you speak to a higher authority. You have certain rights in pregnancy, and if you can prove you are being unfairly victimised because of your condition you will have the weight of the law on your side.

Know your rights

You should know by now that you have a right to be treated fairly and safely in pregnancy. Do try to resolve any potentially problematic situations with your boss or higher authority in your company before you go down the legal route, as it can lead to a lot of stress and heartache. If you feel you have no option but to take a grievance further, we have included a list of addresses of authorities who can help and advise you at the back of the book.

DURING MATERNITY LEAVE

When you go on maternity leave, work will probably be the last thing on your mind, but it's worth knowing what rights you do have during maternity leave, and how you should go about planning if and when you go back to work.

Be aware that your employer is entitled to make 'reasonable' contact with you when you are on maternity leave, and can call or email you if they have an issue that cannot wait until your return; what they cannot do is insist that you come in.

Holidays

While you are off on maternity leave you are still entitled to any paid holiday leave that accumulates while you are away. You can add this to the beginning or end of your maternity leave if you want to extend your time off. What you can't do is carry holiday entitlement over: so if you are due to go on maternity leave in July and your holiday year runs January–December, you need to take your holiday leave at the beginning of your maternity break, as you won't be able to tag it on at the end of the following June.

Benefits

You are entitled to keep any benefits, such as gym membership, as they are a benefit to you and not to the company. If the benefit was for the business – such as a company car or a mobile phone – your employer can legally suspend it for the period of your leave (or loan it to your replacement).

Pension contributions

Your employer must continue to make your pension contributions while you are on maternity leave.

Dismissal or redundancy

If you are dismissed or made redundant it is blatant sex discrimination if it is done because you are pregnant, you are on maternity leave or are absent from the business as a result of your pregnancy, or you are looking after your baby (if they are sick, for example).

Having said that, you can still be made redundant if your employer can prove that the area of the business you work in is closing or your position is no longer viable. If this situation arises you should know that:

- if your employer is making sweeping cuts across the company, he cannot make you redundant just because you are on maternity leave

- if you are made redundant when you are pregnant, you do have additional rights: your employer has to offer you suitable alternative employment in the business if a vacancy exists (even if there is someone else in the company who might be better qualified), and you can start this job (with a four-week trial period) when you return from maternity leave

- if you are dismissed or made redundant during pregnancy, your employer must write to you giving you a full explanation for the termination of your employment and give you your normal notice period, pay in lieu of notice, or redundancy pay if you are contractually entitled to it.

Keeping In Touch/Shared Parental In Touch days

Keeping In Touch (KIT) and Shared Parental In Touch (SPLIT) days are a good idea if you want to stay abreast with what's going on in your organisation or maintain contact with your colleagues. You can spend up to 10 days in your company during your maternity leave without losing your SMP. You are also allowed to work up to 20 SPLIT days without bringing shared parental leave or pay to an end. Remember that:

- you are not obliged to undertake KIT/SPLIT days during your maternity leave, so if you prefer not to go in your employer cannot force you

- your employer must pay you for your time. This may just be for the hours you do, or some companies will pay you a day's wages, even if you only do half a day's work!

- you don't have to do your usual job and these days could be spent training, on a course or at a seminar

- even if you pop in for half an hour it will be treated as a full day for KIT/SPLIT purposes (but not necessarily paid as such – see above)

- you can do them as single days or consecutively

- once you have completed 10 KIT/SPLIT days, if you do any further work you will lose your SMP for the weeks when additional work was undertaken

- you can only do KIT days if your employer is paying you SMP.

Many women find KIT days a useful way of easing back into the working environment after a long break. You could work part-time, eg two days a week, by using KIT/SPLIT days before returning to work. Using KIT/SPLIT days to achieve part-time work for a period may help you and your employer see how well it works, and it may strengthen your argument when making a request to work part-time.

If you do want to take KIT/SPLIT days, make sure that you give your employer as much notice as possible, so that they can plan for your visit and make the day as productive as possible for both parties.

RETURNING TO WORK

Many women are now the main breadwinner in their household and they have to return to work to support their new family. Some also choose to return to work to keep their brain working!

When you are considering returning to work you should know that:

- you need to give your employer eight weeks' notice of your return during your statutory maternity leave. If you don't, your employer can delay your return until the eight weeks have passed.

- if you go back to work before your OML period is up, you are legally entitled to go back to your old job with the same pay and conditions. OML is the first 26 weeks of your entitlement.

- if you return to work during your AML, you should either be given your old job back or a similar position with the same pay and conditions. AML is the last 26 weeks of your entitlement.

- if you are offered a position that you believe to be inferior or with different conditions that you find unacceptable, your company may be guilty of sex discrimination.

Flexible working

For many new mothers, working part time or flexible hours gives them the work/ life balance that they want, and it is always worth investigating the possibility of working fewer or shorter days or working part of the week from home. You might want to sound out your employer during one of your KIT days to give them some notice of what would work for you.

If you or your partner have been working for the same employer for 26 weeks you have a right to request flexible working; legally (and unfortunately), your employer does not have accommodate the request, but they are supposed to give it 'serious consideration'.

Currently, 2.6 million mums are not working in the UK – and for many it is the lack of flexible working arrangements that prevents them from returning to work. Almost 68% of the stay-at-home mums (SAHMs) surveyed in a Digital Mums report said that they would go back to work if flexible working around childcare was an option.

Former career woman?

It's very difficult to say with any certainty how you will feel about your job after your baby is born. One of the fantastic things about maternity leave is that it gives you some breathing space to make decisions about your working life, and gives you time to put the logistics of having a baby and a job in place.

You already know that you are legally obliged to take two weeks off after giving birth, but you cannot yet know how you will feel after you have had the baby: so don't allow yourself to be pressured by your employer, or anyone else, into making a rash decision about your future career. Some women hate being at home, find the day-to-day baby stuff quite tedious and miss the buzz of the office; others adore being at home with their baby and find the idea of going back to the office quite intolerable. Be aware that your feelings can also change as your maternity leave progresses: you might love your freedom from the office at the beginning of your maternity leave, but crave adult company and baby-free conversations by the end.

Some women will feel a loss of identity if they give up their career to stay at home, whereas others will feel so fulfilled by parenting they wonder why they ever worked in the first place.

Whatever you decide to do, there's only one piece of important advice: however long or short your maternity leave is, do try to enjoy it, as you'll never get that time with your baby again.

Child Benefit

Controversial changes to Child Benefit a few years ago has made the system for eligibility pretty complicated depending on whether you are a single- or dual-income household. There's a calculator that is worth filling out on www.gov.uk.

You may have to pay a tax charge if you earn over £50,000, under a 'High Income Child Benefit Charge' – and some couples choose not to claim Child Benefit for this reason.

You'll need to fill out a CH2 form, which is often included in maternity information given out at hospitals or can be downloaded from www.gov.uk. Don't worry if you don't make filling out the form a top priority – payments can be backdated by three months.

CHILDCARE OPTIONS

When you're considering returning to work, one of the biggest considerations you'll have to make concerns childcare. You'll need to decide which type of childcare will work best for you and your baby, and look at the financial aspects as well as what is available to you locally.

Nursery

Advantages

- Your baby will be looked after by a team of qualified individuals.

- Exposure to other babies and young children can build up your child's immune system.

- If a member of staff is ill, your child will still be looked after – it is up to the nursery to arrange suitable care.

- Nurseries are inspected by Ofsted, so you can read past inspections and, just as with any school, get a feel for the strengths and weaknesses of any facility. You can also take some comfort that Ofsted's checking procedures should ensure an acceptable minimum standard of care.

Disadvantages

- Nursery workers can be poorly paid and staff turnover can be high.

- The menu options might be limited.

- Most nurseries only cater for parents working Monday to Friday in office hours.

- If your baby is ill, he won't go to nursery and you won't go to work but you'll still have to pay.

- The cost of nursery care can be high.

Childminders

Advantages

- Many young children like the security of the 'home from home' set-up that a childminder provides.

- A smaller group of children can often mean either a wide variety of activities or activity more closely matched to their needs.

- As with nurseries, childminders are subject to Ofsted inspections; their results are published online and therefore subject to public (especially parental) scrutiny, and an Ofsted inspection should guarantee an acceptable minimum standard of care.

Disadvantages

- Childminders look after many children, not just yours, so they may not have the flexibility to offer as much one-to-one attention as you would like.

- There might be greater opportunities for outings or a wider variety of excursions, but you will probably have to fund these on top of the day-to-day childcare costs.

- If your child is ill, the childminder may not be able to care for him (depending on the other children in their care at the time).

- If the childminder is ill, there may not be scope for any continuity of care – ie you don't go in to work. (In reality, some childminders act as emergency carers for one another and this can work well, but not all childminders offer this facility.)

Nannies

Advantages

- Your baby is looked after in his own home.

- Activities are tailored to your child's needs.

- Everything can work around your baby's existing routine.

- If your baby is ill, the nanny can still look after him.

- As the employer, you get to agree when the suitable opportunities are for your nanny to take holiday days.

- You can nanny-share with friends, neighbours or other parents in the area to save costs.

- Nannies can be employed on a live-in or a daily basis. If you have a decently sized spare room and other suitable facilities (eg an en-suite or room for a TV in the bedroom etc) then you might want to consider a live-in nanny. The overall costs are cheaper. Alternatively, for those who prefer their home to be their own at the end of a long day, a daily nanny could be the answer.

Disadvantages

- If you are the nanny's sole employer, your child may not meet up with many other children unless your nanny is quite gregarious.

- Without other non-family children to play with regularly, your child may take longer to adjust to a school environment and to learn to take turns and fit in with the routine of others.

- You are the employer, so you will need to recruit and interview.

- You will need to draw up a contract of employment and pay employer's National Insurance contributions and tax.

- If your nanny gets pregnant, you will have to pay maternity benefits (although the government refunds these costs) and recruit a temporary nanny to cover the maternity period.

- Not all nannies are Ofsted registered, and some may cost more than others if they have undertaken certain training and have liability insurance.

Help with the cost of childcare

The cost of childcare can be hugely significant. Small wonder then that increasing numbers of retired grandparents are being asked to help with childcare for working parents.

If grandparents aren't an option for you, there are opportunities to reduce the cost of childcare so it's well worth making sure you're up-to-date with everything on offer.

Firstly, it's worth looking into whether you're eligible for the childcare element of Working Tax Credit. The criteria are complicated, but the money available can be substantial and invaluable for helping you back into work. Tax credits are now being merged into the single Universal Credit. Universal Credit will eventually be administered online and these changes will enable greater flexibility for parents whose childcare costs fluctuate from week-to-week, for example, because of irregular work patterns or school holidays. Parents who work less than 16 hours per week will qualify for help with childcare costs through Universal Credit. Go to www.gov.uk/help-with-childcare-costs for more information. In addition, and for everybody else, there is the Tax-Free Childcare scheme.

Tax-Free Childcare

Tax-Free Childcare is a new scheme that gives eligible families up to £2,000 per child towards childcare costs. This is an online system where parents bank their payments. For each £8 a parent pays in, the government will add an additional £2 up to a maximum of £2,000 per year per child. The government website www.childcarechoices.gov.uk allows you to register for the scheme.

Weighing up the costs

Whatever option you decide is the best for you and your child, you need to make sure that the financial cost is less than the financial benefit of you returning to work. This may also be the time to consider working part time.

6
Relationships

We have looked in detail at the practical aspects of your lifestyle in pregnancy, but there are also emotional aspects that are important to cover, because your relationships with the people you love can change quite significantly when you are pregnant. It is as important to feel emotionally well as it is to feel physically well, as there is evidence to suggest that the more relaxed and happy the mother, the easier the pregnancy and birth. We also know that extreme stress is not good for you or your baby, so you need to make sure you take care of your emotional well-being as well as your physical health.

In this chapter we look at the factors that affect your love life during pregnancy and allay any fears you may have. We'll look at the impact your pregnancy and the impending arrival of your child will have on your relationship, and how to make sure you look after your partner as much as you do your baby. Finally, we'll have a look at what having a baby can mean for your relationship with your family and friends, and how to prepare for and cope with these changes.

FOCUSING ON YOUR RELATIONSHIP

Have you ever heard that phrase, 'Having a baby brought us closer together' and thought, 'Are you mad, woman?'. For most of us, there is that wonderful honeymoon period when you find out you are going to be parents, and you are so loved up and fluffy you think you are going to explode. Then the morning sickness kicks in, you start looking and behaving like a spotty teenager and the next thing you know you're having murderous thoughts as he downs his fifth pint and you contemplate driving home without him.

The point here is that pregnancy is not always going to be plain sailing, and your partner is likely to annoy you just as much as he did before – it's just you might be arguing about different things (like names, what football team the baby is going to support, how long your mother is going to stay after the birth, etc).

When you are pregnant, you are often so obsessed with your health and that of your baby it is easy to forget that there is someone else in the relationship and that he is probably as scared/excited/bewildered/fed up as you!

Same-sex partners

Often the road to having a baby isn't smooth if you are in a same-sex relationship. You may have additional worries about bringing up your child – make sure you talk things through with each other regularly. Same-sex couples often recall how important their support networks were to them, during pregnancy and beyond, so do try and find a gay parenting group local to you and join when you feel ready.

SEX DURING PREGNANCY

The embarrassing questions

It's how this journey began, but unsurprisingly sex can be a tad scarce in the months that follow conception and birth. The thing to remember is that you are not alone if you or your partner go off sex during pregnancy. Some women find that while they are pregnant their raging hormones make them feel sexier, and report a rampant sex life during pregnancy. If that's you (lucky thing), enjoy! However, you may find that you are feeling so sick or think you look so much like a whale that sex is the furthest thing from your mind.

However you find your love life developing, you will find that sex is a different thing now you're pregnant. There will probably be several things you might be worried about but are too embarrassed to ask. In this section we'll take you through some of the most common worries women face and give you an honest answer for each.

Will love-making squash the baby in any way?
Your baby is fully cushioned in the amniotic sac and he won't feel anything going on.

Can having sex cause miscarriage?
Unless you have experienced bleeding or have a history of miscarriage, it's perfectly safe to have sex without fear.

Can my partner's penis touch or hurt the baby in any way?

It's anatomically impossible for the penis to make contact with your baby in the uterus due to the angle of the vagina and angle of the uterus. Your cervix acts as a barrier between your baby and your man anyway, so you don't need to worry.

Can my baby be exposed to any infection through sex?

The mucus plug that seals off the cervix prevents bacteria getting through, meaning your baby is not at risk from infection. However, blood-borne infections such as HIV can be transmitted through your blood to the baby. If you have any concerns about blood-borne infections, you should speak to your doctor as soon as possible.

Can I engage in oral sex?

Oral sex is perfectly safe as long as your partner doesn't blow into your vagina. If he blows up there with some force there is a chance that an air bubble could form in your circulatory system, leading to a potentially fatal embolism. However, this is extremely rare, so it shouldn't put you off. It is due to this same risk of air embolism that you should not use jacuzzis during your pregnancy and postnatal period.

Will an orgasm trigger labour?

You may experience mild contractions during orgasm, but they will not be strong enough to bring on labour unless you are ready to give birth anyway. In fact, this is sometimes a recommended way to bring on labour if you go past your due date.

Does the baby know what's going on?

Well, you know now that your baby can hear your voice from quite early on in the pregnancy, so if you happen to be whooping loudly ... In all seriousness, though, you needn't worry that your baby is going to be affected physically or emotionally by your love-making.

Should I avoid sex in pregnancy if my placenta is low (placenta praevia)?

It is advisable to avoid sexual penetration and orgasm if you have a low placenta, as movement of the cervix may dislodge the placenta and cause bleeding. You will be told at your 20-week scan if you have a low placenta and if you should now avoid sex.

The first trimester

If you can't face sex in the first trimester, you are not alone. Many women report that the very thought of sex in the first few weeks made them feel more nauseous than ever. Many women just feel so sick/tired/hormonal that intimate relations don't even come into thought, let alone deed.

It can also be that there are physical aspects of pregnancy that make intimacy uncomfortable, even at this early stage. Many women report that their breasts become so tender, even in the first few weeks, that they couldn't bear for them to be touched. Some pregnant women find they have a heightened sense of smell, which makes it difficult to be physically close to their partner.

If you do feel completely off sex during your first trimester just be honest with your partner about how you're feeling. He'll understand that you're feeling sick/hormonal and won't be offended.

 Words from the professionals

If you have a history of miscarriage, you might be worried that sex in the first trimester could be risky. If you do experience bleeding any time during pregnancy you should ask your GP or midwife whether it is safe to have sex, as obviously you don't want to do anything that could put your baby at risk, however pleasurable.

The second trimester

If your bedroom activities were somewhat limited in the first trimester, things may look up in the second, when you normally have more energy, have got over your sickness and are less anxious and stressed about anything going wrong.

Many women enjoy sex in the second trimester because they actually like their new curvaceous body and feel very womanly; the problem is that their partners don't always feel the same way.

If your partner is unusually reticent to make love, there are a number of reasons why your love life might be lacking at the moment.

- He's frightened that having sex could hurt you or the baby.

- You've gone from being a sexual being to a motherly one, and his instincts might be to protect you and not ravish you at the moment.

- 'He's just not that into you.' Well, not at the moment anyway; many men don't really find big boobs and bellies that alluring, and while you might be embracing all the changes to your body shape he might be quite put off by them.

- The concept of a new life growing inside you is weird enough as it is, and adding sex to the mix just makes it even stranger.

This can be a bit frustrating if you are feeling quite up for it for the first time in months, but don't worry – even if he isn't up for it at the moment the urge will definitely return after the baby is born. You shouldn't take it personally, though: pregnancy is a hugely emotional time for your partner as well as for you, so respect the conflicting emotions he may be feeling.

The third trimester

Things get trickier towards the end of your pregnancy because you get very tired, and there's the logistical aspect of dealing with your bump (the missionary position's going to be out for obvious reasons!). If you do persevere, it's perfectly possible to maintain a happy, fulfilling sex life with some patience, a sense of humour/adventure, and a stack of pillows.

 Words from the professionals

If your waters break early, you experience leaking, have a show (when the mucus plug sealing your cervix comes away) or have placenta praevia, you should seek advice from your midwife before you have sex as it could make your baby vulnerable to infection.

Bring it on, baby!

You've probably heard that making love when your baby is due is a good way to kick-start proceedings. There is some scientific basis for this: semen contains prostaglandin, a hormone-like substance that is said to soften the cervix, and the hormone oxytocin is released during orgasm, which makes the uterus contract and helps to limber up the cervix in preparation for birth. Even if you are the size of a beached whale and sex is the last thing on your mind, you might be surprised to hear yourself asking your partner for a hot session just to test out the theory.

Sex-free pregnancy

You can still enjoy an intimate pregnancy even if you do decide, for whatever reason, that celibacy is the best policy. Obviously there's a number of very pleasurable options open to you, from the sexual (oral sex) to the sensual (body massage). If you can't face full-blown sex, intimacy in the form of kissing and cuddling will make you both feel wanted and loved, and the most important thing is that you still connect with each other physically and emotionally during pregnancy.

It is really important that you keep talking and try to understand why sex is on the back burner. If he doesn't want to make love to you it doesn't mean that he doesn't love you; he might just be feeling scared, weird or worried, and all these emotions are completely natural. If you don't want to make love to him because you are exhausted, feel fat and unattractive or sick, that's also completely normal and doesn't mean you don't care or no longer fancy him. Just make sure that you are open and honest with one another, and take time to be with each other as a couple, without focusing on baby stuff.

Sex after pregnancy

We can't lie and say that the urge to have sex again gets delivered with the baby because it doesn't, and if you are sore and delicate after a difficult birth, the idea of anyone going near you 'down there' is pretty terrifying until everything heals. Slowly but surely, though, you will get through the post-partum baby fug and find your sexual mojo again – well, how else are you going to make baby number two?

OTHER CLOSE RELATIONSHIPS

Relationships with family

Some women are lucky enough to have a very supportive family, but some families have complicated relationships and often a pregnancy can make matters worse.

If you find that your family is proving difficult, try these suggestions to make life easier.

- Be firm with your family if you are worried they are going to take over. If you don't want your mother or mother-in-law to come and stay with you when the baby is born, be firm and say as nicely as possible that you want some time at home alone with the baby (but that you would love them to come and visit for the day).

- Your mum may have seen and done it all before, but parenting styles and opinions have changed. It may take you a while to find your voice, but it's important you make clear that you and your partner will be making decisions for your baby and you may very well choose to ignore her advice!

- Try not to get into any sibling rivalry: there can be tensions when one of you has the first boy or girl in the family, or someone has been trying to get pregnant for ages and you did it at the first attempt. Try to take other family members' feelings into account, as your baby joy might be their baby misery.

Pregnancy can be especially hard if your mum has passed away – you may miss her terribly and desperately want to share this special time with her. Try and remember all the ways in which she was a great mum, and plan to keep family traditions going.

If you have a difficult relationship with your mum, this can also be tricky, as emotions you thought were dealt with may come to the surface. Focus on your immediate family and the future you have together.

Relationships with friends

This one isn't always as simple as it seems. You might be the first one in your social group to get pregnant and suddenly you might be treated like some social outcast. Alternatively, you might be the last one in your gang to get pregnant, and discover that none of your friends is particularly thrilled or excited about your pregnancy because they have seen and done it all before. You might announce your pregnancy just when one of your friends has had a miscarriage or failed IVF attempt and feel incredibly guilty about sharing your happy news, or you might find yourself becoming a baby bore and drive your friends away because all you talk about is your unborn baby. No matter what your circumstances, much like your partner and family, you should try to consider the feelings of your friends, but make sure that you don't let yourself become too stressed or upset by their reactions.

How to sustain friendships in pregnancy

- If there is some tension between friends for whatever reason, remember that most relationships do work themselves out and, even if there is a cooling off during pregnancy, if the friendship is strong you will be able to pick it up at a later date.

- Make time for your friends: if you put all your energy into your baby and your partner, you will miss all the laughs and camaraderie that a girly relationship brings (and boy, you'll need some after the birth!).

- Have a weekend away or a pampering day out. This doesn't have to be hen-style partying in Ibiza, but if you think this will be your last opportunity to go away without a little one in tow, get a group of friends together for some R&R.

- Always make sure to ask your friends what's happening in their lives. Although you're going through a life-changing experience, your friends want to know you still care about their lives and experiences.

- If you find that your old friends really can't cope with the changes brought about by your pregnancy, try making new friends. You don't have to abandon your old ones, but by joining parenting or NCT classes you'll be meeting local women in the same situation, and you might discover a kindred spirit.

GOING IT ALONE

Some women choose to have a baby without a partner on the scene, and other women have this position foisted upon them. Whatever the reason, it is a strong woman who goes through pregnancy without the support of a partner, and hopefully you have a close-knit community of family and friends who can give all the love and help you need. If you are in this position, try making your life easier with a few of these tips.

- Take a girlfriend or family member with you when you buy all your baby essentials, as it can be quite a daunting job to do on your own – and they can help you carry it.

- Shop online and have your bulky and heavy food shopping delivered.

- Enlist help to do anything practical like painting, decorating, or assembling furniture, not only because you might hurt yourself, but because it's also physically difficult to climb a step ladder when you are eight months pregnant.

- Parenting forums can be very supportive: you might also find other local single mums to hook up with.

There may be a silver lining to being pregnant and raising a child on your own: you get to make all the decisions! *You* get to name the baby, decide on the nursery decor and even choose how strict a parent you want to be. There won't be another person giving their opinions or telling you off when you haven't done it the 'right' way.

When your relationship breaks up during pregnancy

Going through pregnancy and birth alone is a pretty daunting prospect, which is why splitting up during pregnancy is really tough.

Pregnancy certainly puts the spotlight on your relationship and can highlight any niggles and imperfections in it; most relationships pull through, but for some couples the strain is too much to bear and they break up.

If you do break up, it's probably worth trying to keep things friendly for the sake of your child. You may not want to ever see him again, but he is your baby's father and hopefully he'll want to have a relationship with the child in the future. He does not have to be named on the birth certificate, but if the split is amicable or you believe that he will continue to play a role in your lives, you can jointly register the birth so that he has Parental Responsibility. If you are not married, the father does not automatically have Parental Responsibility (which is legally defined as 'all the rights, duties, powers, responsibilities and authority which by law a parent of a child has in relation to the child and his property'). If you do not want him to have Parental Responsibility he can go to court after the baby is born to apply for it and ask for access rights too, so it makes sense to try to sort things out now. You'll have quite enough to do coping on your own with a new baby, so if you can get the legal side of things straightened out before the baby is born it's going to be a big weight off your mind. If you need legal help and advice on fathers' rights and responsibilities or single parenting support, there are details of organisations to assist you in the back of the book.

Pregnant and starting a new relationship

You might be single and pregnant by choice, or newly separated from your unborn baby's father, when you meet someone new and 'ping', it's love – probably when you least expected it.

If you are beginning a new relationship, you'll need to consider not only all the usual things, like whether you like him and see a future together; you'll also need to consider your baby. Any relationship you have is going to be a relationship with your child as well, so when you're deciding about whether someone is right for you, make sure you decide whether they're also right for your child.

7

My baby's birth

There's no getting away from it: that baby has to come out one way or another, and it's best to make plans for his arrival in the world (even if it does seem a very long way off). Keep a fairly open mind about proceedings, but do give some consideration to the type of birth you want and where you want to have the baby – after all, it might go exactly as you hope!

In this chapter we'll look at the kinds of things you need to consider in your birth plan and how best to prepare yourself for the big day.

CHOOSING WHERE TO HAVE YOUR BABY

There are generally three options when it comes to choosing where you give birth: at home, in a midwife-led birth centre or on a hospital labour ward. Some hospitals do not have midwife-led units and some do not offer home birth; it is something you need to find out before you book at a hospital. Some women will not be offered the choice because they have a medical or pregnancy complication, so the safest place is a labour ward, but they should be informed of the reasons why this is being recommended.

> **Words from the professionals**
>
> People who come in with a fixed idealistic birth plan often don't get the birth they planned for and feel disappointed, as if they have failed. The best situation is a woman who knows how she'd like to give birth but has considered – and is informed of – all possibilities so that if anything diverts from her plan she still feels in control and understands why it has happened.

It's well worth researching the options available to you, because your choice may well affect the type of birth that you have. Check out the website www.which.co.uk/home-birth if you want some impartial advice on where to give birth locally. You don't have to stick with your decision, though; if you want to change your mind and opt for different care, you are entitled to do so. Sometimes it may mean going to a different hospital to deliver, however, especially if the hospital does not have a birth centre or offer home births.

Consultant-led hospital unit

The consultant-led unit is where you will be advised to give birth if you have any complications or concerns in pregnancy, if you are being induced, if you are having a Caesarean section or if you would like to be able to have an epidural. You will be in a room of your own and have a midwife looking after you. There will also be doctors caring for you.

Hospital units can vary enormously – from shiny and high-tech to crumbling and Dickensian – so if environment is important to you, there's a possibility you will have to travel to find what you want. Do bear in mind that although you can choose to give birth outside your local area, journey time is an important consideration because babies can arrive unannounced and unexpectedly, even first time around. Also, after your delivery, the midwives who visit you at home will come from the local hospital, not where you delivered.

Pros

- There is an obstetrician on call, should you experience complications during delivery.

- Hospitals are best equipped to deal with medical emergencies.

- You can have an epidural, should you need one, as there is an anaesthetist on hand 24 hours a day.

- If your baby is born early or with problems, a paediatrician can be present at the baby's birth, and there will be a specialist neonatal unit where he can be cared for.

- If you have problems after the birth, you will stay in hospital and be cared for by doctors and midwives.

- If you have a high-risk pregnancy, you will be seen by a consultant at the hospital.

Cons

- Hospital wards can be rather grim, unfamiliar places.

- You may not have met the midwives who'll deliver your baby.

- Your partner may not be able to stay with you if you are on the postnatal or antenatal ward at night, but can stay with you when you are in labour.

If you are lucky you might find that your hospital has both a consultant-led maternity unit and a midwife-led birth centre, so you can choose between the two as your pregnancy progresses.

You might want to take a hospital tour to find out what sort of care is on offer and what facilities are available (although this might be a virtual tour to prevent spread of infection). Even if you have no choice, it's still useful to find out as much as you can about the hospital, because it's possible that the next time you see the maternity ward will be when you are in full-blown labour, and the location of the catering facilities or the loos will be the last thing on your mind. Look at the hospital's website or in your hand-held notes, as you may be pleasantly surprised that most of the answers are there!

Private rooms

Many women are generally very pleased with the level of care and attention they get from their local NHS maternity unit, but like the idea of having a private room after the birth. Often referred to as amenity rooms, they are only suitable if you and baby are well enough to be alone, so are not suitable immediately after a Caesarean section. When you take the hospital tour, ask if any rooms are available, how and when they can be booked, and how much they cost, as prices will vary enormously. You won't get private care, treatment or special meals, though, and some new mothers have reported that they felt quite isolated in them, so take a look before you decide to go for one; if your birth has gone smoothly you could go home the same day and won't need one.

Midwife-led units/birth centres

Midwife-led units (also commonly known as 'birth centres') provide a sort of halfway house between hospital and home births. The rooms are usually more homely than consultant-led delivery rooms and, as the name implies, there are no doctors for you or for the baby.

The difference between birth centres and consultant-led units is that the former are staffed and run by midwives. If the birth centre is attached to the consultant-led unit, there are doctors on hand if things go wrong and you can easily be transferred to the labour ward if necessary. If the birth centre is a stand-alone centre away from the hospital, you will be transferred by ambulance with the midwife to the consultant-led unit if complications arise. Birth centres are gaining in popularity and around 10% of women in England delivered in one last year. Check out www.which.co.uk/birth-choice if you think this sort of care is for you.

Words from the professionals

What's the standard procedure for going to hospital when you think you're in labour? Phone the hospital when you think you are in labour, and the midwife will either give you advice over the phone or tell you to come in to be assessed. When you come in, you and your baby will be assessed and you may be examined to see if your cervix is dilating. If you are in early labour – before 3cm dilated – you may be given advice, such as a recommendation to go home for some rest and return when your labour has progressed. If you do not want to go home, you may remain in the antenatal ward to wait for labour to become fully established; it is generally best to go home as women tend to cope much better and can relax more in their own home. You may well be in a bay with other women on the antenatal ward, which many women don't enjoy, and would prefer some privacy. It is not until you are admitted to the labour ward and in established labour that you have your own room and your own midwife.

Midwife-led units are normally more low-tech and homely – for example, one in London has fibre-optic lights and funky bean bags and looks more like an average teenager's bedroom (albeit rather more sparse and tidy) than a room you'd expect to give birth in, which is precisely the appeal of these centres.

You should be aware that you will only be accepted for care at a midwife-led unit if your pregnancy is low risk: that is, if you have no complications and are expecting a healthy baby. Your age may be a factor with some centres too, and for most, being overweight will be an exclusion. If you have gestational diabetes or high blood pressure, or if you know your baby is going to be born early or have health problems, you will usually need some input from a doctor, so you will probably need consultant-led care. The midwives are trained in life-saving and resuscitation techniques should your baby need help, and if you are in a birth centre joined on to a consultant-led unit there will be obstetricians and paediatricians available in an emergency. If you are unsure, ask your midwife or doctor where they think you should deliver your baby.

In many hospitals the main delivery suite also has birthing pools, balls, etc. So if there is a reason for you to be on the delivery suite to have your baby you can still have many of these natural relaxing techniques.

Pros

- A relaxing environment to give birth in. Rooms are usually equipped with mats and bean bags to give birth on.

- Your partner may be allowed to stay the night with you after the baby is born, space and schedule permitting.

- You'll be provided with equipment to facilitate natural birth, such as birthing pools, birthing balls, etc.

- Statistically, you have a lower chance of having an assisted delivery (and you would need to be transferred out for this).

- You are less likely to tear or have an episiotomy (when they have to cut your perineum to help the baby out), as labours are lower risk. See page 230 for more on episiotomies.

- You may be offered complementary therapies such as aromatherapy or acupuncture to make the birth a less painful and more relaxing experience.

- You may have your own private en-suite room after delivery.

- You will have access to Entonox (gas and air).

Cons

- If the pain becomes unbearable, you won't be able to have an epidural at a birth centre.

- You will have to be transferred to hospital if you or your baby get in trouble during labour or after delivery.

- You can't have a Caesarean section at a birth centre.

- If your baby needs special care after birth, he will have to be transferred to hospital.

- If the unit is a stand-alone birth centre, it may be some distance from a hospital and transferring could take time. If it is a birth centre joined on to a consultant-led unit this is a lesser issue. Around 22% of first-time mothers do transfer to hospital or the labour ward from a birth centre, so if it happens to you your midwife will be used to this and will make the transition as smooth as she can.

Women who use birth centres report very high satisfaction with the standard of care they receive, and experts believe that if women have good one-to-one care during labour they are more likely to have a straightforward birth.

Midwife-led units are a very positive development in the provision of maternity services, and are definitely worth considering if you are low-risk and the idea of a natural birth appeals.

Words from the professionals

What happens if there are no free beds available when I go into labour? It's very rare that there are no beds for women to deliver in, but if this is the situation, then the unit will have an agreement with a hospital close by in which you will be able to give birth. While it is very unusual for this to happen, it can undoubtedly cause a certain amount of anxiety if this situation arises, so do ask this question when visiting your midwife-led unit. Each hospital closely monitors how many women are due each month, so it can manage its staffing and beds.

Home births

In England, around 2% of births take place at home. The popularity of home births has seen a change over the decades: in the 1960s one third of all births were at home, but by the late 1980s, less than 1% were home births. This percentage then rose steadily to a peak in 2008 at 2.9%. These rates vary in other UK countries – 2.7% in Wales, 1.5% in Scotland and 0.4% in Northern Ireland – but all of these figures hide local peaks and troughs, so check your local hospital. In some parts of the country, the percentage of women choosing to have a home birth is as high as 11%. A study from the end of 2011 showed that for women having their first baby, home birth resulted in three times as many complications, but the absolute risk was still low.

Some women love the idea of giving birth in their own home in a relaxed environment, while others like the security of having doctors on hand. The choice is totally your own, and you should just make sure you consider all aspects of this option.

You *should* be offered home birth as an option, although a recent survey revealed that only 57% of pregnant women were offered it by their midwife at the booking appointment. However, only women with no complications and a normal singleton pregnancy would be offered a home birth, which perhaps explains this statistic. If you have complications such as pre-eclampsia, are expecting twins or your baby is breech, your midwife will encourage you to have a hospital birth as the labour needs additional monitoring.

The appeal of a home birth is obvious but it is not without its risks, and you should weigh up the pros and cons and have a good chat with your doctor and midwife before you decide it's the birth option for you.

Pros

- You give birth in a familiar environment surrounded by the things (and people) you love.

- You can be tucked up in your own bed straight after the birth.

- You have complete privacy.

- You don't have to share wards or bathrooms with anyone.

- You have two midwives looking after you and it's likely that you'll know one or both of them from your antenatal appointments.

- The midwives will also stay with you for the duration of your labour, so you won't have the change of shift that can blight a hospital labour. The two midwives will relieve each other if it is a long labour.

- You can recover in the relative peace and quiet of your own home.

Cons

- You'll probably only be able to have gas and air at home (although some midwives can administer the drug pethidine).

- If anything happens during labour that the midwife can't deal with, you'll need to go by ambulance to hospital.

- If an emergency arises during labour, there will be time spent travelling to the hospital that could at best be uncomfortable, and at worst could endanger your life or your baby's life.

- You might miss the security of 24-hour midwifery care that you'll get in hospital after the birth.

You should be aware that some health professionals don't support the idea of home births for first-time mothers, and other health authorities won't sanction one on the grounds of cost. If you really want to have one and you are coming up against opposition to the idea, you can always book a private midwife to look after you in the last weeks of pregnancy.

PRIVATE CARE

If you can afford it, there are plenty of private care options you can choose during pregnancy, birth and beyond. Be aware, though, that going private won't guarantee a better, safer or more comfortable birth. You might get more attention, more pleasant surroundings and nicer food, but these do not guarantee safer or better midwifery or medical care. Every birth is different and there are only so many factors determined by the location.

Independent midwives

Independent midwives are fully qualified midwives who have chosen to work outside the NHS in a self-employed capacity, and look after you before, during and after the birth. Some women choose to hire an independent midwife because they want continuity of care throughout their pregnancy; others take on an independent midwife because they will facilitate a 'natural' or home birth if a woman wants one but has been advised against it on the NHS, or it is not available locally. Recent statistics from the organisation Independent Midwives UK showed that nearly 80% of deliveries under independent midwife care were 'normal', ie the births had no medical intervention.

Independent midwives are fully regulated in the same way as midwives in the NHS, and must adhere to government rules and guidelines. They are also subject to annual inspection visits and equipment checks.

How much do they cost?
A lot will depend on where you live and the package of care you choose, but ballpark figures show that, on average, independent midwives charge between £2,000 and £4,000 for their services. Normally this has to be paid in full by week 36 of pregnancy.

Pros

- An independent midwife will build up a relationship with you before your baby is born, which may result in a better birth outcome.
- She may help you to have a home birth if you have been advised against one by the NHS.
- She will stay with you throughout your pregnancy, birth and for an agreed period afterwards, so you have continuity of care.
- She works alongside the NHS, so that you can still have all your scans and tests done in hospital.
- She is trained to deal with emergencies and will stay with you if you need to be transferred to hospital.

Cons

- Independent midwives do not have personal liability insurance, so you can't sue them if something goes wrong. Although midwives seem to want insurance, insurers aren't keen to provide it at the moment as there are too few in the UK to make a profit.
- If you have to be transferred to hospital she will stay with you as your birth partner, but will let the midwives and doctors at the hospital take over your midwifery care.
- If the NHS has declined a home birth, there might be very good safety reasons for this, so be sure you aren't taking risks.

For more information on having an independent midwife, visit imuk.org.uk.

Doulas

The word *doula* (pronounced doola) derives from a Greek word meaning servant or caregiver, and a doula will do just that during birth: attend to your needs and help you emotionally and physically, but not clinically. She is not qualified to provide medical care, but can support you as a primary or secondary birth partner. The doula philosophy is to 'mother the mother', so you get lots of support during birth.

If you want to hire a doula, she will normally meet you a couple of times before the birth and then will be at your side during the big event. She can also follow up with postnatal care if you want more help.

What does she do during birth?

A doula might help you with your breathing, relaxation techniques, help you get into comfortable positions, and offer continuous nurturing support. She can also be your advocate and tell the health professionals your desires for the birth.

Pros

- If you are by yourself a doula will be your primary birthing partner, instead of you labouring alone.

- She will be known to you, and that may be important if you don't know your midwife at the birth.

- Studies have shown that having a doula present reduces the need for medical intervention and can shorten labour time.

- She can focus on you while the midwife focuses on the safe delivery of the baby.

- She can help you after the birth, which is useful if you do not have support from family or friends. She will often help you around the house or look after other children so you can have time to care for your baby.

Cons

- It's important that you get on with your doula, as she has to work closely with you, your partner if they are present, and the midwife during labour, and you may struggle to find someone you like locally.

- Postnatal support is extra and will be a minimum of £10 an hour. Doulas normally want three-hour bookings as a minimum, and travel expenses may also be charged.

How much will it cost me?

An experienced trained doula will charge between £250 and £500, depending upon where you live, her travelling expenses and experience. Trainee doulas cannot charge more than £200, according to their governing body.

How do I find one in my area?

An excellent online resource is www.doula.org.uk, which has a handy section of questions you can use to vet a prospective doula to see whether she is the right one for you.

Private hospitals

The most exclusive (and expensive) option is to go for consultant- or midwife-led care in a private hospital or birth centre. There are also consultants and midwives that provide private care in local NHS hospitals, so it may be worth researching the private options available in your local hospital if this is the sort of care you think you may want.

How much can I expect to pay?

It really depends on the level of care you want and where you want to give birth. You can find 'birth only' packages countrywide for around £850; private care in an NHS hospital at around £5,000; and care at a private hospital from £8,000 (but that's just for a midwife-led package – a consultant is going to set you back considerably more).

What will I get for my money?

It varies depending on where you have decided to give birth and what facilities you have paid for, but can feature the following.

- Full maternity packages often include four detailed scans, antenatal appointments, routine blood tests, 24-hour telephone support, and postnatal checks, along with complementary therapies and private GP visits.

- A 'birth only' option means you have NHS care up until labour. You then give birth in a private facility and usually stay for around eight hours afterwards. If all is well, you are discharged into the care of your community midwife. Usually this type of birth is not recommended for first-time mothers, and it's easy to see why: if something does go wrong you may rack up thousands of pounds in additional fees, so you need to ask yourself whether the benefits outweigh the potential disadvantages.

- You can opt to have your own dedicated consultant or midwife that you see at every antenatal appointment – but bear in mind it can cost twice as much to have consultant-led care rather than midwife-led care.

- You will have an en-suite room of your own after birth – the degree of luxury will obviously depend on the hospital.

- You may well get better food than standard NHS fare, and you may even be able to order a little tipple to wet the baby's head.

- Your partner may be able to stay with you overnight and visiting times and numbers may be more relaxed.

- You should be able to expect a better level of postnatal nursing care.

Bear in mind that you may find that the private hospital does not have the same array of immediate emergency staff available if there is an unexpected problem. Check who is on call at night and whether there is an intensive care unit for your baby or you.

WRITING A BIRTH PLAN

The benefit of making a birth plan is that it does focus your mind on the type of birth you would ideally like; it also forces you to consider things you would rather avoid during birth if at all possible. Critics of birth plans say that they are about as useful as a chocolate teapot, as every birth is different and no one can predict what is going to happen. Many women find that decisions they'd made before labour go out of the window once they are faced with the pain of contractions – there's many a story of women opting for epidurals, when they'd expressly said before that they wanted a natural birth. Although in the end the birth may be nothing like the one you imagined, your birth plan can really help you to focus on what you do and do not want, and prepare for what can happen. The other benefit of a birth plan is that it does encourage you to confront the possible issues that can arise during birth, which is beneficial if you are in a state of denial about the whole thing and hoping the baby will just magically appear at the end of nine months.

Remember that midwives and doctors will always aim to discuss options with you as the labour unfolds, so you don't have to foresee every permutation, nor worry that you or your birthing partner will be excluded just because you haven't written something down.

The most important thing to remember is that you have to keep an open mind and be flexible about the whole thing. There is no benefit in putting 'I refuse to have any medical interventions' or 'I must have an epidural', because you don't know how your labour will progress and how you are going to cope.

If you are not given a printed birth plan to fill in, you can make your own using the questions outlined below to guide you. Make sure it is legible and preferably typed. If your partner is present at the birth, make sure he knows what you wrote on your birth plan, and discuss it with those providing your antenatal care too – particularly if there's something in your personal circumstances that might have a significant bearing on how you want your baby delivered, or your personal care during labour.

Questions to consider:

- What are your ideal pain relief choices?
- Are you happy for students to attend the birth?
- What position do you want to give birth in?
- What birthing aids do you want to use?
- Does your partner wish to be present at a Caesarean section?
- Do you want an anaesthetic for a Caesarean section, or an epidural?
- Do you want the baby delivered onto your chest or to be cleaned up first?
- Does your partner want to cut the umbilical cord?
- Do you want an injection to contract the uterus and deliver the placenta?
- Do you want your baby to have a vitamin K injection?
- Do you plan to breastfeed?
- Do you wish to feed straightaway?
- Do you wish to be cared for by women only?
- Do you need an interpreter?

If you have strong feelings about any of the above, it might be useful to use the phrase, 'I should like to avoid X and Y, but if my health or that of the baby is in danger I consent to having medical intervention to deliver my baby safely'.

You might also like to state what kind of birth you are hoping for, ie 'natural' if that is your wish. (See page 164 for more on natural births.)

YOUR BIRTHING TEAM

While you are thinking about your baby's birth, it is useful to consider who you want to be present at the birth. Until the 1960s, men were actively discouraged from being in the delivery room, but these days around 90% of fathers attend their child's birth.

Do check your hospital or birth centre's rules about the number of people allowed to attend the birth; if you have a home birth your midwife might allow a few more people in the room, but in hospital you are unlikely to be allowed more than a couple.

If you want your current partner to be your birth partner, it's handy if he knows what to expect during the birth. It can be surprisingly difficult to persuade a man to pick up a pregnancy manual, as even the most excited of prospective fathers are terrified by the idea of birth and don't want to read about it. Do ensure that he has a rough idea of what he is letting himself in for, though, because it can be very upsetting seeing someone you love in such pain or having a medical procedure you weren't expecting. Many pregnancy units run classes that have sections aimed specifically at prospective fathers, so they are worth attending.

If he doesn't want to read a weighty medical tome on pregnancy and birth you could give him this chapter to read, or buy him the bestselling book *Pregnancy for Men* by Mark Woods (White Ladder, 2018).

Eight things your birth partner should know

- It may be stating the obvious, but childbirth is incredibly painful and it is likely that you will scream, rant or swear. Most women do!

- You may do quite odd things to cope with the pain, like bite your hand or make strong, guttural noises.

- Prepare him for possible birth interventions: explain what ventouse and forceps delivery are and why they might be used (see pages 228–231 for more information).

- Explain that sometimes you can't get a large head through a small hole, so occasionally women tear or need an episiotomy. The reason it's good to prepare him is that sometimes you will need stitches after birth – this can be alarming if he thinks your future sex life is literally getting stitched up, but more importantly he might be left holding the baby if your midwife needs to do some minor repairs on you after birth.

- Tell him about the kind of birth you are planning. Many men probably still imagine we all give birth lying down with our legs in the air, and he might think you really have become deranged with pain if you start wandering around or squatting in preparation for an active birth.

- There is a lot of blood, and if he is at all squeamish he probably should stay away from the 'business' end. It's not uncommon for men to faint during childbirth, and even if they don't actually faint, it can get pretty messy down there, so it's best to prepare him.

- Explain what happens to the baby after birth (see page 233), and that your work isn't done until you've delivered the placenta.

- Give him the opportunity to say if he wants to cut the umbilical cord.

Useful things your partner can do as a birth supporter

Before you go into labour it can be helpful if your partner takes on the following tasks.

- Stops drinking alcohol in the run-up to your due date so that he can drive you to the hospital, rather than having to call a taxi or a nearby friend or relative.

- Works out the route to hospital and does a dummy run before your due date to get timings right.

- Keeps an eye on roadworks and closures. He won't want to deliver the baby himself in the car if you don't make it in time.

- Works out where to park when you get to hospital and makes sure he has enough money to pay and display if necessary.

- Puts essential numbers into his phone so he can call or text family and friends. And, of course, he'll need to make sure his phone is fully charged!

- Takes enough cash to pay for magazines, treats and drinks. If your labour is prolonged you will need entertainment and sustenance.

- Takes responsibility for putting your birth bag/luggage in the car (many a bag has been left at home in the excitement).

- Makes sure he knows how to fit the baby car seat. You might be home in 12 hours with your baby if you are lucky – so take it with you when you head off for hospital just in case.

While you are in labour your partner can provide the following support.

- Make sure he has read and understood your birth plan in case you are not able to state your preferences during labour.

- Give him some idea of how active you want him to be in the birth. Some partners are physically supportive as well as emotionally; you might want to lean on him while you're pushing, or you might want him to just hold your hand or stroke your hair.

- Make him aware that the birth cannot be controlled, and that just because you wrote something on your birth plan doesn't mean you can't change your mind. You don't want him 'helpfully' reminding you that you said you didn't want an epidural when you are screaming for an anaesthetist because you can't bear the pain.

- Give him a job to do if you think it will keep him calm: it might be feeding you ice chips, getting you drinks (if you're allowed them) or spraying you with water mist to keep you cool. If he is a bit of a control freak or the dominant one in your relationship, try to make him understand that *you* need to dictate what happens during the birth.

The professionals

You will (hopefully) have plenty of help and care from a midwife, and possibly a doctor if labour isn't progressing as it should.

If continuity during the birth or knowing who is going to deliver your baby is important, we have already outlined the options available to you to try to get the midwifery care that you want. If you give birth in a large urban hospital, it is very possible that you will not have previously met the midwife who delivers your baby. If you are in this situation, there's not much planning you can do in advance, but it is a good idea to prepare yourself for what might happen so it doesn't throw you on the day.

Firstly, there is the issue of shifts. In an ideal world, you would have the same midwife with you throughout the birth, and some of them are such dedicated professionals that they do stay on to help you if you are in the final stages of labour. The hospital staff have rotas for a reason: to ensure there is a even level of care at all times and that staff don't get dangerously tired.

It is entirely possible that you may not form a bond with your midwife: midwives are like anyone from any walk of life – some people you get on with and others you don't – but at the end of the day, as long as they are competent and deliver your baby safely, it's really not worth getting stressed about bonding with them, unless you do feel that your health or that of your baby is in jeopardy. If you are really unhappy with your midwife you should quietly tell the midwife in charge of the shift about your concerns: she may be able to change staff around if it is just a personality clash.

Don't get worried if you have a student midwife on hand either: this is quite common in teaching hospitals, and it can be very positive having an extra pair of hands helping to look after you.

The key to having a happy birth is not to worry too much about the things you can't control. If you love your midwife or hate her, if you have one midwife or 10, it really doesn't matter as long as you and your baby come out of it physically and emotionally intact.

Be prepared for everything and anything

You can make things easier for yourself by being completely up to speed about what is likely to happen on the day. Don't decide to read the chapter on giving birth as your first contractions start; you need to have a good idea of the stages of labour and, even if it does make scary reading, know all your pain relief options and learn what could go wrong (even though it's unlikely). The reason this is important is that you may have to make decisions during labour, and if you are ill-informed you may make the wrong one and end up with a birth you won't want or enjoy.

PLANNING FOR A NATURAL BIRTH

Definitions of a 'natural' birth vary, but in general it means a labour and birth without pain relief (apart from gas and air, which still counts as 'natural') and without intervention (such as forceps or surgery). For many women this is the ideal birth – to deliver in the way nature intended – and indeed it is the way that many women in the world give birth, particularly if they don't have access to hospital facilities.

The issue of natural birth is an emotive one, with its advocates arguing that if women were left to their own devices with a supportive midwife, there would be far more natural deliveries than we have at present.

Plan for a natural birth by all means – there are plenty of good reasons why you should – but please don't feel that you have failed if it doesn't happen. Just remember, your goal is to deliver a healthy, happy baby who won't give two hoots about how he arrived in the world. There is always that cliché that if men had to give birth they would have invented a way to make it painless by now; well, to an extent they have – it's called an epidural, and if you want one, have one. You don't go to the dentist and say, 'I'd like an extraction without the anaesthetic because I want to feel the pain,' and the same should apply to childbirth. You are no less of a woman or a mother if you want every drug and intervention going.

Pros

- Studies show you are likely to suffer less postnatal pain and have a faster recovery.

- You may have a higher sense of awareness during the birth.

- You may bond better with your baby as a result of a rewarding birth experience.

- Your birth may be more enjoyable if you are in a more relaxing environment like a birth centre.

- There are lots of nice relaxing techniques like water baths and massage to help you.

Cons

- There's no getting away from it: birth can hurt, a lot, and many women have no idea what their pain threshold is like until they have a baby.

- Some women only increase their stress levels by worrying that they need to persevere and have no pain relief.

How to increase your chances of a natural birth

- Statistically you are more likely to have a natural birth if you give birth at home or at a midwife-led birth centre (but this is at least partly because you have a low-risk pregnancy).

- If you're giving birth in hospital, make sure that your desire for a natural birth is written clearly on your birth plan, and make sure your birth partner knows what you want so he can speak up during labour.

- Sign up for NCT classes or active birth classes. Their focus is normally on low intervention or natural birth, and any classes on relaxation and breathing are good preparation for labour.

- Consider a water birth. Studies have shown that women who spend even part of their labour in a birthing pool are less likely to need pain relief such as pethidine or an epidural, and there's some evidence that shows it could reduce the likelihood of tearing or the need for an episiotomy. Some women choose to give birth in the water, while others use the birthing pool for pain relief and relaxation but give birth 'on dry land'. Even a warm bath can have therapeutic qualities during labour. If you are giving birth at home you can hire a birthing pool; and many standard maternity units in hospitals have them now too, so it's worth asking when you do your hospital tour. Check any weight/size restrictions. If you are overweight, you may not be able to give birth in a birthing pool, as a hoist may be needed. If you are interested in a water birth then discuss the practicalities with your midwife.

- Look into the possibility of using alternative methods of pain relief such as hypnotherapy, acupuncture, aromatherapy, massage, TENs machine and breathing techniques (see pages 176–179).

- Have a woman as a delivery partner. Research shows that a female companion in the delivery room can improve your chance of having a birth without intervention. If you think your baby's father might be a bit upset if you tell him he can't come in, then ask your mum, a friend or hire a doula to come as well.

- After 37 weeks, if he's not there already, encourage your baby into the right position prior to birth – ie head down: do this by getting on all fours to allow your baby the space and gravity to move. If the baby is breech, you may be offered external cephalic version to turn him round to head down, or a Caesarean section.

HAVING AN ACTIVE BIRTH

Active birth became popular in the late 1970s, when pioneers of this type of birth recommended that women should be free to move around spontaneously during labour, and adopt upright or squatting positions to give birth. Fans of active birth believe that it makes birth less painful, easier, and more efficient. For many women, it works (you have gravity on your side for a start); they also believe it is a more natural way to deliver as it is universally and culturally adopted the world over.

However, over 50% of women in the UK still deliver lying on their backs on a bed, with critics saying that it is easier for the health professionals to manage the labour if the patients are lying down. There can be patient-led reasons too, though: some women get quite embarrassed squatting or kneeling half naked in front of people they don't know and want the security of a bed and sheets where they can have some degree of modesty, and some just feel that lying down is right for them.

If you like the idea of an active birth, there are lots of websites where you can read up about it and decide if it is the birthing style for you. If you want to give it a go, make sure you put it in your birth plan and talk to the midwife about it at the start of your labour.

PLANNED CAESAREAN SECTION

If your midwife suspects you will have to have a planned Caesarean section, you will normally see a doctor to discuss the pros and cons and work out what is best for you and your baby. Caesarean sections account for around 23% of births in this country, and if you know in advance you are going to have one it is called a 'planned' or 'elective' Caesarean section. Around 37% of all Caesarean sections in the UK are planned or elective. This type of Caesarean section will be recommended if the health professionals believe in advance that it will be safer for you or your baby to deliver this way.

There are a number of reasons why your obstetrician might want to pencil in a Caesarean section for a birth.

- If you have placenta praevia.

- If your baby is breech (bottom first) or transverse (lying sideways), and attempts to turn him have failed. It is possible to have a breech baby vaginally, but for some women a Caesarean section is considered safer.

- If your baby is too small (intrauterine growth restriction) or already distressed.

- If you are suffering from pre-eclampsia (although vaginal birth is often encouraged).

- If you are expecting twins and the first is NOT head down there are more likely to be complications and a Caesarean section might be recommended. Do keep in mind that it's not unknown for one twin to be born vaginally but for the second twin to be delivered by Caesarean section. Many women do give birth to twins vaginally (around 50%), but if you are expecting more than two babies it is almost certain you will be having a planned Caesarean section.

- If you have had two or more Caesarean sections before or if you had complications in a previous vaginal delivery that could recur.

If your consultant recommends that you have a planned Caesarean section, it will be because he has the health and safety of you and your baby in mind. It is quite a major operation with an extended recovery period, so it is not something that he will suggest without careful consideration. It must be explained clearly to you why this procedure is the best option, and you should have plenty of opportunities to discuss the options. Don't be afraid to ask questions, and even ask for a second opinion if you are not sure – no one will mind! While you may be tempted to research other options, please try to avoid the temptation to use the internet – it is so difficult to find reliable information that you can trust, and usually there will be circumstances unique to you that will only be apparent to someone talking to you.

Pros

- The birth will be quicker.
- The birth itself should be less painful.
- You know when you are going to have your baby.
- For planned deliveries many units now offer a 'gentle' Caesarean section, with a quiet, calm, low-lit environment, allowing you to see baby as he is born and to put him on your skin as soon as possible.

Cons

- Recovery time is longer and you have to spend longer in hospital – your baby stays with you, though, and you are supported by midwives and nursery nurses to care for your baby.
- Statistically, they carry an increased risk of complications (see opposite).
- You might feel cheated as you didn't give birth as nature intended (but you shouldn't).
- You are more likely to have complications in your next pregnancy.

Also, do remember that things change – you may be booked in for a Caesarean section if your baby is breech, but he may move at the last moment. Your baby's position should be regularly monitored in case he turns head down at the last moment and you can attempt a vaginal birth.

Elective Caesarean

The latest NHS guidance is that, on safety and cost grounds, Caesarean sections should not be performed on maternal request alone. However, it is quite obvious that some women do have elective Caesarean sections for non-medical reasons, and some private clinics are prepared to carry them out. On the NHS, if there is no physical reason for a Caesarean section but you still feel that it is what you want, talk to your midwife and doctor as early as possible in the pregnancy. They should try to understand why you want a Caesarean section, and may be able to give you a clearer picture of the pros and cons. They may suggest input from a perinatal mental health psychologist if they feel you have a birth anxiety condition.

Caesarean section fact file

Having a Caesarean section is not the easy option when it comes to giving birth; there are many risks associated with them, which is why doctors don't recommend them on a whim. The complications associated with Caesarean sections can mean:

- you have an increased risk of excessive bleeding and needing a blood transfusion

- you have an increased risk of developing a blood clot (thrombosis) in your legs or lungs (see page 64) and are more likely to need to give yourself once-a-day heparin injections for 10 days or six weeks afterwards to try to prevent one

- you are more likely to suffer abdominal pain

- you are more likely to be re-admitted after birth or to have further surgery

- you are more likely to get an infection (wound, uterus, urine, chest or blood for starters!) and will be given preventative antibiotics as the operation begins

- you may have complications in future pregnancies

- baby is more likely to be admitted to a Special Care Baby Unit (SCBU)

- there is a 1% chance your baby's skin will be cut during the operation.

The points above show that having a Caesarean section is not a stroll in the park, but do remember that most women who have a Caesarean section don't suffer any long-term effects, and the safe delivery of your baby should override any worries about possible complications of the surgery.

Fear of giving birth

Although you might be over the moon about your pregnancy and thoroughly excited about becoming a mother, it may well be that you are frightened of giving birth, but you're too embarrassed to admit it.

Don't worry: there's not a first-time mother in the land who isn't frightened of giving birth – you are certainly not alone.

The problem for all pregnant women is that the fear of giving birth is the fear of the unknown. You have absolutely no idea how your labour is going to go, and that's why the thought of it can be so scary. You also worry that there might be something wrong with the baby that you'll only discover once it's born. The best advice is to read up as much as you can about giving birth and prepare yourself for every eventuality; it won't necessarily influence the outcome of your birth, but it might help you make informed decisions on the day.

Tokophobia

Tokophobia is the extreme fear of giving birth and was only recognised as a medical condition in 2000. It is thought to affect as many as one in seven women. If you think you have tokophobia, ask for counselling or hypnotherapy to help you overcome it. If you are truly traumatised by the idea of giving birth vaginally, it is essential that you speak to a doctor as early as possible, who may refer you for a psychological assessment; depending on the circumstances, you may overcome the fear and aim for vaginal birth, or you may need a Caesarean section, but this is best decided in conjunction with experts in the area.

MULTIPLE BIRTHS

If you are having twins, you will usually have consultant-led antenatal care, including more scans to check that each baby is growing normally, more checks for pre-eclampsia and gestational diabetes and more discussion about the options for delivery. Women having twins are more likely to develop problems during their pregnancy, although of course not everyone does! These might include:

- exaggerated symptoms of 'normal' pregnancy such as thrush, urinary frequency, heartburn, tiredness, backache and pelvic discomfort

- anaemia – most women with twins should take an iron and folate supplement routinely, to supply enough for both babies and themselves

- pre-term delivery, baby or babies smaller than expected, pre-eclampsia, gestational diabetes or thrombosis in your legs.

It is entirely possible to give birth to twins vaginally, and this is often recommended. But your doctor may recommend that you have an elective Caesarean section to give birth if, for example, the first baby is not coming head first or if the pregnancy is complicated in some other way.

Occasionally during a vaginal twin birth, the first baby is born vaginally but the second has to be delivered by Caesarean section because he's in the wrong position or an emergency arises, so you should be prepared for that eventuality.

If you're having more than one baby you should also know the following.

- Twins are usually born earlier than single babies, probably because they stretch the uterus more. As a result of this they are smaller and lighter on average than singletons. A twin pregnancy is considered full-term at 37 weeks, not 40 weeks like single pregnancies.

- If you are having a multiple birth there will normally be more people in the delivery room, including (possibly) a paediatrician for each baby, an obstetrician or two and a couple of midwives. The anaesthetist is usually in the vicinity too.

- If you have twins, you will be recommended to deliver in a consultant-led unit.

- You are quite often induced around 37–38 weeks if you have not gone into labour before this, and often it is recommended that you have an epidural to help with the safe delivery of each baby and in case a Caesarean section is necessary.

PREMATURE BIRTH

If your baby is born before 37 weeks the birth is considered to be premature. About 7% of babies are born before 37 weeks, including about 1% born before 28 weeks.

Sometimes you will know in advance that it is more likely to happen; for example, if you have a medical condition that means you are unlikely to carry until full term, if you are having more than one baby, or if you have had trauma to or operations on your cervix. There are several exciting trials going on at the moment trying to predict and prevent pre-term birth, so don't be surprised if you are asked to take part. If you do know that your baby is likely to be born before 37 weeks, you might want to visit the SCBU, or meet some of the staff who will care for him – ask your doctor or midwife about this.

Sometimes you just go into labour spontaneously: you may start contracting or the membranes may rupture prematurely. This is more common if you have vaginal bleeding or if you have a raised temperature for a prolonged period, but sometimes it has no identifiable medical reason at all. If you have any bleeding after 24 weeks or if your temperature won't settle with paracetamol, then you should **always** be checked out at the hospital.

It is often not clear if symptoms are pre-term labour or due to something else. You may be offered a vaginal swab test called fetal fibronectin. A low result means pre-term delivery is unlikely to be imminent.

Travelling after 24 weeks

The possibility of pre-term delivery will also mean you have to reconsider travelling abroad after 24 weeks. If your pregnancy is normal, it is unlikely that you will deliver pre-term, but if it does happen while you are out of the country, the logistics of looking after yourself and a newborn baby in a neonatal intensive care unit overseas are worth considering carefully – is the trip really worthwhile at this stage of pregnancy? Can someone else go? Can it wait until after you deliver? If you do travel, please check your insurance policy to make sure it includes cover for you and for your baby.

What risks are associated with having a premature baby?

Many babies born pre-term are completely healthy and well. However, babies who are born before they are full term are more likely to develop health problems because they haven't had the chance to fully mature in the uterus. You should be aware that:

- in the early days they may have problems breathing, feeding and regulating their own body temperature
- they may be more prone to infection when they are first born
- they are more likely to develop problems post-birth, such as anaemia and jaundice
- some are more likely to have longer-term problems, such as issues with their hearing or eyesight, and some may have neurological problems such as difficulty or a delay in walking or talking, or difficulties with cognition, co-ordination or concentration.

There is no doubt that babies born very early are more likely to suffer short-term health problems but the good news is that current survival rates are improving.

- Recent figures show that around 20% of babies have a chance of survival if born at 23 weeks, although many have long-term disabilities.
- At 25 weeks they have a 67% survival rate, and around half will have a disability.
- At 32 weeks they are likely to survive without any significant health problems.

If you go into labour early you may be given treatment to temporarily halt contractions, giving you time to get to a hospital with specialist facilities for premature babies. The doctors may also offer you two injections of steroids, which help the baby's lungs to mature and so reduce the chance of severe breathing problems by 50%. These steroids also reduce the chance of the baby having a brain haemorrhage by 50%, and improve his chance of survival. Therefore, although it may sound a bit scary to be offered steroid injections, these are in fact very well proven to help your baby. Latest research shows that an infusion of magnesium sulfate started four hours before you deliver prematurely can improve your baby's health by protecting his brain.

Tommy's has an excellent and free book *Having a Premature Baby* that you can order online at www.tommys.org if you are affected by pre-term birth.

 Words from the professionals

If you are bleeding, having regular contractions, your waters have broken or are leaking or, if you think you may be in labour for any other reason, you should contact your delivery unit immediately – or, if you are really concerned, call an ambulance and go straight to your local maternity unit.

PAIN RELIEF OPTIONS

We have looked at the types of birth you can plan for: now we can consider your pain relief options, so you can research them and note what you think you might like (or not like) on your birth plan.

There's no doubt that giving birth hurts. But it is very difficult to generalise about it because everyone's coping mechanisms and pain thresholds are different. If you find the pain unbearable, there are several options to make you more comfortable, and our advice would be to take them!

Just remember one thing: however bad the pain, a lot of women go on to have another child – so despite the terrible agony, you may soon find yourself willing to give it another go!

Entonox: gas and air

Entonox is a mix of 50% oxygen and 50% nitrous oxide, and is administered through a mouthpiece or mask that allows you to breathe in the gas during a contraction.

When can I have it?

In theory you can have gas and air at any time during labour or birth, but let your midwife be your guide. If you are in early labour and find you need pain relief, this probably isn't the best choice.

Is it any good?

It's not the most powerful form of pain relief, but it can certainly help you deal with contractions for a while. It can take up to a minute for the effects to kick in, so it's best to take it when you feel a contraction coming on, rather than start it in the middle of one. You need to remember to stop using it at the height of the contraction, so that it wears off as the pain ends – that way you won't feel too spaced out in between contractions. Partners and midwives can be quite useful for gently dissuading you from gulping down more than you really need!

You can also use it at a home birth, in the birth centre and in the birthing pool.

Any side effects or anything else I should know?

Gas and air undoubtedly creates a sort of 'high' that can make you feel woozy, drunk or slightly out of control. However, this feeling wears off minutes after you stop inhaling. It can also give you a dry mouth and can sometimes make you feel nauseous. It is not harmful to you or your baby, and probably the worst thing about it is that your birthing partner will try to wrestle it off you for a go!

TENS machine

A TENS (transcutaneous electrical nerve stimulation) machine is a little box which emits electrical pulses through four wires and four sticky pads, which you fix to your back.

The theory is that it intercepts the pain signals to your brain and stimulates the release of endorphins, the body's natural pain-relieving hormones. There are dials so you can control the frequency and intensity of the pulses. You need to start off low and increase them as the contractions get stronger.

When can I have it?

As early as you like, although be aware that it takes up to an hour for your body to respond, so you need to get it on in good time. You are best to start using it at home as soon as labour starts. You are likely to need help from your birth partner or midwife to put the wires on because it is a bit fiddly to do by yourself. You'll probably want to ditch it towards the end of labour, because the wires will become a nuisance and TENS machines aren't normally capable of dealing with really strong contractions.

Does it work?

Opinions vary: they seem to work for some women and not for others. They can be a great distraction from pain and help you feel in control as you press the buttons when you feel a contraction coming.

Any side effects or anything else I should know?

There are no side effects when using a TENS machine, but you can't use them in a birthing pool for obvious reasons; electricity and water don't mix! You also can't have a back massage if you have the pads on and you can feel a bit constrained by all the wiring. Beware turning them too high: you can get a pulse so strong it gives you a bit of a shock. TENS machines aren't routinely available in all maternity units, but if your hospital has a stash you might be able to borrow or hire one. If not, you can hire them from places such as Boots. They cost around £20–£30 to hire and £50–£60 to buy.

Painkilling drugs (pethidine, Meptid and diamorphine)

These painkilling drugs (also known as analgesics) are usually administered by injection into your thigh or bottom, or occasionally into a vein in your arm. Midwives are able to give you these drugs, so there is no need to wait for the OK from an obstetrician or anaesthetist.

Pethidine is the most commonly used painkilling drug. Pethidine is great when you feel Entonox is not quite enough, as it just gives slightly stronger pain relief and can be used along with gas and air. It can be given in some birth centres and some midwives will give it at home births. It is the next strongest thing after Entonox, but it is not as effective as an epidural.

Meptid is a strong painkiller, and it doesn't make the baby as sleepy as pethidine (see below). Diamorphine is not used in many maternity units now as pethidine and Meptid are much safer and more effective.

If you find that the painkilling drugs are not strong enough, you can still go on to have an epidural after having pethidine or Meptid.

When can I have them?

You can have these painkilling drugs at any time until you are close to the pushing stage. If you have these drugs too late in labour they will not be effective, as they take about 30 minutes to take effect; they can also make the baby sleepy just before he is born, which could make him take longer to start breathing and slow to feed. If there are severe problems with the baby's breathing at birth following pethidine (which is rare), there is an antidote the baby can be given to stop the pethidine effects.

Does it work?

Some women find these drugs very effective; others don't. Even if they don't take the pain away, they might make you feel more relaxed between contractions.

Any side effects or anything else I should know?

These drugs can make you feel drowsy, dizzy or sick: you will usually be given an anti-sickness injection with them to reduce the chance of you getting nauseous. If you have too much or are given them too late, they may hang around in your baby's system for a few days and could make him sleepy, slow his breathing or make it difficult for him to feed. Allergic reactions are rare, but do ensure your medical team are aware of any known allergies.

Epidural

An epidural is an anaesthetic injection into the lower part of the back, which numbs the nerve supply serving the uterus and cervix and gives complete and quick pain relief. Some hospitals offer mobile epidurals (lower dosage injections) that give pain relief but don't numb the legs so much (but you're still not normally allowed to walk around).

When can I have it?

As a rule of thumb, you can have an epidural as soon as you are in established labour (see page 223) or you feel the pain is more than you can deal with. If you are being induced you may want to have it around the time that the Syntocinon (oxytocin) hormone drip is started. The effect lasts several hours, and it can either be topped up as you require or maintained using a constant infusion – each hospital has a slightly different approach but patient-controlled administration of the epidural solution is increasingly popular – you control how much you have and when, and this results in greater satisfaction and less medication being used. Most women will keep it working until they have delivered; it used to be said that you should let it wear off when the time comes to push so that 'you can feel what you are doing' – while this may suit you, it is certainly not encouraged, since it can be really hard to deal with the pain again *just* when you need to focus on pushing. Modern epidurals often allow complete pain relief, but the sensation of pressure is maintained so you can feel a contraction coming and push without pain.

Does it work?

In a word, yes. However, there is also the possibility that it will take only partially – some women have relief on one side of their body, and have to be positioned on a bed to assist gravity and 'move' the medication to both sides.

Any side effects or anything else I should know?

It can completely numb your body from the waist to your toes and you won't be able to walk around. If you have an epidural you will need a drip in your arm in case your blood pressure drops and you need to be given fluid quickly. Your baby will also be constantly monitored. You will need a catheter (a tube going into your bladder) to help you urinate, as you won't be able to feel if your bladder is full or not. Some women experience severe headaches, shaking, backache or fever after having one.

You need to have an anaesthetist present to site the epidural into your back and give you the first dose. This can take up to 30 minutes to be fully effective. The midwife will then give the rest of the painkillers into the epidural site when they are needed, or you can do it yourself by pressing a button on a patient-controlled analgesia pump. Most maternity units have an anaesthetist on staff 24 hours a day just for maternity cases; however, if he is busy in theatre you may have to wait for him to become free, and occasionally the baby will arrive before the anaesthetist! In some hospitals you might struggle to get one in the middle of the night; you also won't get one in a birth centre or at a home birth. If you think you may want an epidural it is worth asking in advance if there is a 24-hour anaesthetic service.

Epidurals are fantastic at taking away the pain of childbirth, and you shouldn't feel that your birth experience is inferior because you chose to have one. Giving birth should be a joy and not a competition, so if you can't stand the pain any longer you should definitely ask for one. At the end of the day there are no medals for bravery.

Alternative pain relief

If drug-taking and button fiddling is not your thing, there are other pain relief options you can explore. Make sure you note them on your birth plan if you want to give them a go.

While these might have been considered genuinely 'alternative' a few years ago, you may find that more and more midwives are open to the idea of different methods of pain relief, and many already practise them. Some women find that they can be very successful when used in the early stages of labour, particularly if you combine a couple of them. Other women find they don't work at all. The trick is to consider them and give them a go by all means, but if you find they are not working for you then ditch them and try something else.

Acupuncture

You are probably already familiar with the ancient Chinese therapy that involves the insertion of fine needles into various points in the body. It is said to stimulate the energy channels and release endorphins, which are the body's natural painkilling hormones. It is also thought to be quite effective at inducing labour that is overdue. There is some evidence to show it can reduce labour pain intensity, increase patient satisfaction and limit use of pharmalogical analgesia including epidural use. In some European countries midwifery-delivered acupuncture in labour is common and now some UK hospitals are beginning to offer this – so ask your midwife. If your local hospital doesn't offer it, you can find a qualified private practitioner through the British Acupuncture Council.

Aromatherapy

Aromatherapy is the use of natural essential oils that are said to have a positive effect on the body and mind. These oils can be diluted and used in massage, inhaled via a burner or vaporiser, or put on a hankie or pillow as droplets. You should avoid putting them directly on your skin or into the water of a birthing pool; however, they can be used in a bath. Some oils are unsuitable for labour, so you should check with a trained aromatherapist before you use them, or do some careful homework on the subject. It's unlikely aromatherapy will do much to improve the pain of labour; however, the back massage might, and it may aid relaxation in the early stages. It can stimulate more effective contractions and, if nothing else, will make the delivery room smell good!

Breathing techniques

Slow, rhythmic deep breathing can help you relax during labour, and you're more likely to cope with the pain if you can relax into it rather than fight against it. Breathing also helps you conserve your energy and boost oxygen supplies to you and your baby. Here are some tips:

- Focus on a two syllable word (relax is actually a good one): think 'reeeeee' as you breathe in slowly and 'laaaaaax' as you breathe out again.

- Try counting as you breathe in and out, or breathing in through your nose and out through your mouth.

- Get your birthing partner to help you and join in with your breathing exercises.

Be aware that breathing techniques might help you in the early stages, but may not do the job when the pain is so bad that breathing becomes a labour in itself. Pregnancy yoga classes are often effective at teaching breathing techniques.

Heat therapy

Some women find heated pads useful during labour, in the same way that many of us put a hot water battle on our tummies to alleviate period pain. You might find that it does a job for you in the early stages of labour but probably won't hack it towards the end.

Conversely, if you find labour makes you feel very hot, ask your birth partner to wet some cool flannels and apply them to your eyes, forehead or neck. Refresh them often and suck on ice chips to cool your mouth, but do not apply ice directly to bare skin, as it can stick to you and cause burning.

Hypnobirthing

Some people believe that you can take the pain of childbirth away, or distract yourself from it, using hypnosis. Hypnobirthing is based on the theory that fear causes great tension and that in turn leads to pain, and it's believed that if you put your mind into a state of deep relaxation then the pain will go away. If you want to learn these techniques, you'll need to find someone qualified to teach you and then practise them before the birth. You can also buy CDs that teach hypnobirthing skills.

An NHS study into the effectiveness of hypnobirthing in helping women give birth without painkillers has shown no difference in the use of epidurals, but possibly a reduction in postnatal anxiety.

Massage

Massage is another technique that is supposed to release those natural endorphins by putting pressure on the body's energy channels. Massage definitely boosts relaxation and gives you a sense of wellbeing, especially if lovingly applied by a willing birth partner, so it might make you feel emotionally better even if it doesn't do much for you physically. Shoulder massage is effective to relieve tension, and a lower back massage is useful for trying to alleviate the pain of contractions. Bring along a small wooden massage tool for your partner to use if his hands get stiff. Slow, rhythmic strokes or circles, firmly applied with the fingers or the palms of the hands, are most effective, but you can be the judge and tell your partner what is working for you. Many women can't bear to be touched during labour, so warn your partner beforehand that you may rebuff him on the day, even if you have enjoyed massages throughout the pregnancy.

Visualisation and vocalisation techniques

You can look into visualisation techniques where you 'see' each stage of labour (which can make it easier to cope with), or vocalisation, when you sing, chant or grunt to relieve the pain: you may baulk now, but on the day you might do anything to take the pain away!

Reflexology

Reflexology involves massaging particular points of the feet, and is said to work in a similar way to acupuncture by tapping into the body's energy channels and releasing naturally occurring painkillers. You'll need to find a qualified practitioner to help you if you want to try it during labour.

Water

Many women report that a birthing pool of warm water can be a very relaxing, effective method of pain relief. Widely available in maternity units and birthing centres, you can also hire one if you are having a home birth. If you are giving birth in a hospital where a birthing pool isn't available, you may be able to wallow in a warm bath instead (as long as someone is with you). Many women who have had successful water births claim they are comforting, and others said they helped make birth a 'calm' and 'peaceful' process. Remember that you won't be able to have anything stronger than gas and air in the birthing pool, so if you want to hit the drugs you'll have to get out.

8
Baby shopping

This chapter gives you a rest from all the medical info and deals with the fun stuff – like shopping and planning your baby's nursery.

In this chapter we take you through your baby essentials and desirables, and we'll also give tips on budgeting and how to get the best deals.

Some women are superstitious during pregnancy and don't want to go shopping until the final weeks, but as one in 10 women delivers prematurely, there is a slight chance that you might go into labour and not have all the things you need. It also makes sense to start your baby shopping at the start of the third trimester, when you are still quite mobile and probably not as tired as you might be at the end of your pregnancy.

Of course, due to the wonders of the internet you could, in theory, do all your baby shopping online. Our advice is to do your research online and then try to check out the key items in store, because you might want to properly test just how easy that drop-catch cot side is to release, or feel the weight of your favoured buggy or test how foldable it is.

ESSENTIAL BABY CLOTHES

The first piece of advice is: don't spend a fortune on newborn outfits. You will invariably get lots of baby clothes as gifts so, without sounding cynical, let family and friends indulge your baby while you stick to the practical items.

Babies should wear natural fibres like cotton, as they 'breathe' better. Babies are not so good at regulating their body temperature, so they shouldn't wear man-made fibres that could cause them to overheat. Cotton jersey is probably the best fabric for your baby essentials because it is soft to the touch, won't irritate your baby's skin and is stretchy, which is useful as you will be taking these clothes on and off all day. If you are prone to allergies and think your baby might have sensitive skin, organic cotton baby clothes are widely available.

Babygros, sleepsuits and vests

If your baby is born in the colder winter months, you will need seven long-sleeved vests and ideally around 14 babygros or sleepsuits (long-sleeved body suits with feet attached). If your baby is summer-born it might be more sensible to buy 10 short-sleeved vests and 10 babygros.

Because newborns often vomit up some milk and new mothers can be slow at nappy changing (don't worry, you'll soon be a pro), it's useful to estimate using two babygros during the day. You'll spend a lot of time nappy changing and feeding, so it makes sense for your baby not to be trussed up in too many fiddly layers. Keep it simple with these vests and babygros.

Your baby may very well live in a babygro during the day for a while, and you may only bother getting him 'dressed up' for visitors or outings. There's nothing wrong with that!

A hat

Your baby will need a hat – or most likely two because invariably one gets lost or forgotten somewhere. Babies need to wear hats to keep them warm and also to protect their heads from the sun.

If your baby is summer-born, try a soft jersey beanie to keep him warm (they are also very easy to get on and off) and a sunhat to protect his head and face from the sun's rays. A winter-born baby might need a soft fleece pull-on and maybe a wool one if you have a knitting granny (make sure it's not scratchy, though).

A cardigan

You need to dress your baby in layers when you are going out, and a cardigan is ideal: because they are short they don't interfere with nappy changing and are reasonably easy to get on and off. Again, if you are given hand-knitted cardigans, be sure the wool is good quality and not scratchy.

A coat or all-in-one suit

If you know you are going to be out and about doing a lot of walking, consider buying your baby a padded, waterproof all-in-one suit. These are a bit fiddly to get on and off, but it does ensure that he is evenly covered and warm. If your baby is mainly going to travel by car, a coat or lightly padded jacket should suffice, but don't put him in heavily padded suits because they can interfere with a car seat's protective qualities.

Mitts

Babies have quite sharp fingernails, and despite your best efforts to cut them, they can cause quite a lot of damage to delicate newborn skin. Mitts do, however, fall off very easily and many babygros now have fold-over sleeves to do the same job.

Bibs

It's useful to buy some towelling or soft jersey bibs because babies dribble milk or posset, whether they are bottle or breastfed. If you pop a bib over his clothing, it obviously stops you needing to change a complete outfit.

Swaddle blanket

You might want to consider a swaddle blanket for your baby. Research has shown that babies who are swaddled (wrapped quite tightly) in a piece of fabric settle better because they feel secure like they did in the uterus, although you must be careful not to let your baby overheat. You can use a shawl or a specialised, slightly stretchy, swaddle blanket. Some people advise that you stop swaddling at around four to six weeks, because babies need to be free to move around to help their motor development.

Practical tips

When you're choosing clothing, try not to be seduced by pretty prints or cute designs only – bear in mind that you will potentially have to change these outfits several times a day for many months! Therefore, outfits with awkward buttons, tight necks and fiddly elastic will soon be abandoned at the back of the wardrobe. Go for poppers, soft fleeces and common-sense designs.

Equally, look at the washing labels. You'll be handling mountains of washing – some babies can go through several outfits a day. Hand-wash and dry-clean-only garments are a bad idea, unless they're for a special occasion. Look for materials which wash well, don't pill and keep their shape.

Remember to wash all items of clothing in a mild detergent before you put them on your baby – clothes come with various starches and chemicals in them, which may irritate your baby's skin if you put them on straight from the shop.

In terms of colour and design, avoid clothes that will look tired, washed out and ruined once they've been through the wash several times. Choose darker colours or fabrics with prints to disguise stains. And look for fabrics suitable for the 'dry and fold' technique – no need for the iron!

PRACTICAL KIT

Pushchair/pram/travel system

You could probably write a whole book on this subject alone, so we will only cover the options available and let you research and decide what is right for you.

Before you buy, consider the following.

Where you live/your lifestyle

- If you live in the country and plan to take your baby on rough terrain, you might want a sporty three wheeler that can tackle hills and bumps with ease.

- You might live somewhere so remote that you are going to spend most of your time ferrying your baby around by car; if that's the case, you'll need a buggy that will fit easily into the boot.

- If you live in a congested urban area, you might want something reasonably compact, as pounding the pavements can be quite tricky with a big buggy.

- Are you planning on having more children in the near future? If you are, you might want to consider one of those pushchairs that convert to a two-tier configuration, so you can accommodate two children, with the baby on the top and the toddler below. Considerably slimmer than the traditional double buggy, many parents find these are a good solution for a growing family.

- Do you plan to travel a lot with your baby? If so, you might consider investing in both a proper pram and a 'holiday' buggy. A fold-up umbrella-style pushchair is a good investment for air travel, as it can usually be folded once you get to the aircraft.

- Do you want to get fit with your baby? You can buy jogging buggies that are specially designed to let you run and push your baby comfortably at the same time.

Your budget

You can spend anything from £20 to £2,000 on a pushchair, so it is important that you set a budget.

Your baby might start walking at 12 months, but the reality is that you may still be pushing your tot around in a buggy four or five years from now, so you want to buy something you know is going to last. The pushchair is probably the most important purchase you will make, as you'll probably be using it every day and it will be subject to much more wear and tear than something like a cot. For this reason, you might want to spend as much as you can possibly afford (although make sure it ticks all the boxes as far as your requirements go).

New research shows that while parents may be happy to use second-hand clothes and toys, the vast majority want to buy brand new prams and buggies. At the top end of the market, the must-have Bugaboo, chosen by royal parents William and Kate, the classic Silver Cross favoured by celebrity mums such as Madonna, Victoria Beckham, Liz Hurley and Sarah Jessica Parker, and the ever-popular iCandy fruit-inspired models have gained almost cult status.

Travel systems
In essence, a travel system is a pushchair that is compatible with an infant rear-facing car seat, and often comes with a carrycot that you can attach to the chassis.

Pros

- If your baby is asleep you can simply unclip him from the car and clip him onto the pushchair frame, without the need to wake or unstrap him.
- This is a convenient and sometimes economical way of buying the car seat, carrycot and pushchair all in one.
- You can have your baby facing you.

Cons

- Your baby will grow out of the carrycot within months.
- You will need to buy another car seat once your baby is around a year old and weighing over 10kg (22lb).
- The chassis can be heavy and difficult to fold in some designs.
- These systems are not cheap, ranging from around £200 to £1,000.
- Not all infant car seats are compatible with travel systems, so you should check before you buy if purchasing separately, or buy everything as a complete package.

Lightweights
If you are looking for a buggy that is easy to fold and light to push, there are many models on the market. Most have the traditional umbrella-type fold, but in the last couple of years some exciting new designs have come onto the market. Improvements in design mean that they have become more comfortable in recent years, with more attention to padding and detail in the seat area.

Pros

- Light to carry.
- Traditionally easy to fold.
- Often more compact than other types of pushchair.

- Useful if you live in a flat and have to fold and carry up stairs.

- Good for urban living where space is tight.

- Usually have a carry strap or handle.

- Good budget option if cash is an issue.

Cons

- Some are not suitable for newborns.

- Some models are quite basic and don't have sophisticated suspension or braking systems.

- Not good for bumpy countryside walks or travelling on sand.

- May seem the cheapest option, but you'll bump up the price if you buy all the optional extras.

Sporty pushchairs/three-wheelers

If you have a fairly active lifestyle and can see yourself taking the baby on long country walks, jogging or taking a stroll in the sand dunes, you'll need a pram that can cope with all terrains. Traditionally, this type of pram was called a three-wheeler, but there are more four-wheeled versions coming onto the market. They're not just for country dwellers, though; they'll be as happy pounding pavements as hiking over hills.

Pros

- Flexible – you can use them wherever you are.

- Easy to manoeuvre.

- Suspension is normally really good.

Cons

- Can be bulky when folded. Sometimes you need to take the wheels off if you are attempting to put it in the boot of a small hatchback.

- Can be quite heavy.

- Can be expensive.

Pushchair buying checklist

- Do your research on the internet and then find a local stockist that has all the styles you are interested in. We cannot stress too much the importance of actually handling the pushchair to see if it is comfortable, folds easily and manoeuvres the way you want it to.

- Accessories are very important, but check what is included in the price, because extras can really bump up the cost of a basic model. A rain cover is essential because you'll need to keep your baby dry, and a sunshade and shopping basket/storage are desirable.

- Make sure the handles are easily adjustable, as your partner might be considerably taller than you and what is comfortable for you will not necessarily be comfortable for him.

- Check it will fit easily into your car boot when folded; you don't want to have to take the wheels off to wedge it in.

- Look at the seat positions on your favoured models; can it lie flat, for example? This is useful when your newborn is sleeping most of the day because it will be more comfortable for him.

- Are the brakes foot operated or operated from the handle? Test the brakes to see if they are easy to access.

- For a smooth, comfortable ride, the pushchair should have good suspension. You can test this by pushing down on the buggy; if it bounces back in one smooth movement then it's probably a goodie.

- How easy is it to handle? Can you get it through narrow gaps with ease? This is useful if you're going to be using it for shopping.

- If you are going to need to carry it up stairs (for example, if you live in a flat), or use public transport frequently, look at lightweight models.

Car seat

If you have a car, you will need an infant car seat, and if you are going to bring your baby home from hospital in a vehicle, you need to know how to fit it properly before the baby is born. Hospitals *will not* release babies without a car seat if they are travelling home in a vehicle.

Things you should know

- There are two types of infant car seat: Group 0, which is from birth to 10kg (22lb); and Group 0+, which is from birth to 13kg (28.5lb).

- All babies must be rear-facing until they are 15 months old. The reason for this is that it is much safer for your baby if you have a crash, as the force of the impact is more evenly distributed if he is rear-facing.

- If your baby is going to travel in the front seat and you have airbags in the front, they *must* be deactivated as the force of the airbag could kill your baby if it inflates. If you cannot turn the airbags off, your baby must be strapped in the back.

- Most newer cars have an ISOFIX-compatible system, an internationally recognised safety standard that was launched with the backing of car seat manufacturers. ISOFIX seats clip into a base that stays in the car and are supposed to be safer and easier to use.

- If your car is older or doesn't have ISOFIX, you will have to use the traditional seat belt method.

- You should not buy second-hand car seats because you don't know their history. If they have been in a prior accident or have a hairline crack, they could severely compromise your baby's safety if you are involved in an accident.

- Not every car seat will fit every car, so make sure you try before you buy; many stores such as Halfords offer a car seat fitting service if you go to their larger outlets with space outside for your car.

- Babies up to six weeks old should spend no more than 30 minutes in a car seat at a time, and older babies should preferably spend no more than two hours a day in a car seat, as research has shown that babies have low levels of oxygen in their blood if they sit in the same position for hours at a time.

You don't need to worry about the safety aspect when you buy an infant car seat from a reputable baby goods manufacturer, because it will have been subjected to rigorous tests before it came on the market. There are, however, certain features that offer more protection, make the chair more comfortable, or the seat more user-friendly, so it's worth doing some research before you buy.

Car seat buying checklist

- Does your favoured model actually fit in your car? Try before you buy!

- If safety is an issue and you have the ISOFIX system in your car, it's worth buying a compatible car seat. A recent survey showed that only 4% of ISOFIX car seats were incorrectly fitted, whereas a whopping 60% of traditional car seats were not fitted properly.

- How heavy is it? The car seat you choose may look lovely, but if it weighs a ton it won't be easy to get in and out of the car with a chubby baby inside.

- Does your baby fit in it? Very small or premature babies are too small for normal car seats and require specialist car cots to travel in. Likewise, if you're purchasing a seat for a child who has outgrown one already, make sure the weight restriction goes high enough.

- Does it have a head hugger? These removable padded supports are good for giving your newborn extra support and protection and for making him feel more secure.

- How deep are the safety wings? The deeper and more padded the 'wings' of the car seat (the sides by your baby's head), the better the protection.

- Can you take the cover off and wash it? Useful if the baby is sick all over it or has an explosive poo.

- How adjustable is the handle? Some handles go forwards as well as back, so that the car seat can become a rocker inside your home.

- Does it have additional safety features? All car seats come with a three-point harness, but some new models have five-point harnesses.

- Does it have a reclining feature? Some models on the market allow your baby to lie flat, which is more comfortable for him.

- Is it buggy-compatible? It may fix to the frame of your chosen pushchair. Most car seats are compatible with their same-brand pushchairs, but the Maxi Cosi fits most pushchair options.

Sling/baby carrier

Sometimes it is more convenient to just pop your baby in a sling or baby carrier than to go out with a pushchair. You don't have to buy one new, however; it's the perfect item to borrow if you have a friend who has one lying idle. There are several types of slings: there's the traditional fabric type that you can tie in a variety of ways; there's the papoose type where your baby lies vertically against your chest; and there are some on the market that start life as a papoose and can be converted to a hip carrier once your baby gets bigger.

Babies usually have to be a minimum weight before you can use a carrier. You can face him out when his neck is strong enough, which lets him see the world on the go. You must make sure there is sufficient hip support – your baby's legs should be in a 'W' shape, like a frog, and not dangling from the hip sockets.

Pros

- You can keep your baby close to you, and the sound of your heartbeat can be reassuring to him.

- This is a very convenient way to transport your baby because you have your hands free.

- With a baby carrier, you can turn the baby face out when he's old enough.

Cons

- A recent study in the US showed that there is a danger of suffocation if the baby is curled up in the sling and his oxygen supply is restricted (more likely if you use the fabric type and the baby is cocooned rather than upright).

- If you have a bad back or a particularly heavy baby, you might find it puts too much strain on your lumbar region after a few months, or even weeks.

- It can be tricky to put the baby into the papoose if you are on your own.

Sling or carrier buying checklist

- How long will you be able to use it? Does it convert for use with a toddler?

- Is it well padded, with protection for your baby's head?

- Can the baby face inwards and outwards?

- Is the fabric breathable or can your baby get too hot?

- Can you use it from birth? Some companies recommend that you use them after one week or after a certain weight.

- Can you wash it?

Changing bag

In theory, you can manage without a changing bag, but we normally succumb to buying one because they are designed to make nappy changing on-the-go as quick and efficient as possible.

What you need to know

- It helps if your changing bag can function as a handbag as well as a nappy bag (meaning you don't have to carry two bags around), so it makes sense to buy one that you like the look of, as you will be using it every day.

- There are some really cool designs on the market, so do some research before you buy.

- If you don't find anything you like, go the DIY route; as long as a bag is roomy, has handles you can sling over the buggy (or is a backpack), you can buy the components separately to create the functional bag you want.

Changing bag buying checklist

- Is the bag wipe-clean? That butter-soft tan bag may look gorgeous, but if you accidently get some baby poo on it you'll be traumatised (patent would be a great choice).

- Does it have somewhere special to stash your mobile phone, keys, wallet, etc? Many changing bags have key clips, phone holders and special pockets, so keep an eye out for these features.

- Does it have insulated pockets to keep milk or food chilled? Useful if you are going to be out all day.

- Does it have a fold-up padded changing mat? Obviously you need to be able to wipe this clean, but it also helps if there is some padding in case you have to change your baby somewhere unforgiving, like on a hard floor.

- Does it have a removable bag for soiled clothes or nappies? Desirable but not essential, although it does help if you have a separate bag you can wash inside the changing bag for stained clothing, or nappies if there's no disposal bin nearby.

Steriliser

If you know that you are not going to breastfeed, it makes sense to buy a steriliser before the baby is born. There are basically two different types: electronic steam sterilisers and microwave sterilisers, but both types create steam to sterilise the bottles. Many retailers sell starter packs with bottles, teats and other accessories included, which can work out cheaper.

What you need to know

- Some sterilisers keep the items sterilised for 24 hours. If you are working or have other time pressures, this feature will be a godsend because it means that you will only be sterilising once a day.

- Some models are quite big and cumbersome, so if space is tight in your kitchen, you might have to find a small model or look at the microwave options that tend to be smaller.

- Sterilising times can vary between four and 10 minutes, so if time is precious or you are worried you might have to sterilise in the night, go for one with a quicker time.

Steriliser buying checklist

- How many bottles will it hold at once? If you have twins or your baby turns out to be hungry you'll want a bigger one.

- Does it only work with the same brand bottles? This is important if you wish to use BPA-free ones (see page 192) and they are not compatible with the steriliser.

- Are you likely to travel a lot with your baby? Choose a model that is compact; a microwave version is probably the easier option.

Understanding BPA

There is some concern over Bisphenol A (BPA), which is present in plastic in some baby bottles in the UK. Exposure to BPA has been linked to breast cancer and there is a possibility that it can have an effect on your baby's reproductive, neurological or immune systems. Canada has recently withdrawn from sale all baby bottles containing BPA, and an EU ban on BPA in baby bottles came into effect in June 2011. In July 2012 the USA also implemented a ban. Read the latest research and make an informed judgement on whether you think the risk is significant enough to opt for BPA-free bottles; they are widely available and should be clearly labelled 'BPA free'.

Muslins

Muslins are absolutely essential when you have a newborn. Every baby tends to regurgitate some milk after feeding or winding, and the idea of the muslin is to protect your clothing from that vomited milk.

What you need to know

- They are going to be in the wash all the time as they are going to get covered in stains, so buy in bulk.

- You can find them in lots of colours.

- Extra large ones can double up as swaddle blankets.

Baby hygiene and grooming

Experts recommend that you wash your baby's face and bottom with just water for the first few weeks (a practice known as 'top and tailing'), so there's no need to buy any baby bubble bath yet.

If you want some in the cupboard in readiness, make sure you buy baby-specific products, as chemicals in some adult soap products may irritate your baby's delicate skin. If you have sensitive skin or are worried about chemicals there are lots of organic baby products on the market.

Things you need (or might want)

- **Cotton wool.** You'll need this for cleaning faces and bottoms (although obviously not with the same piece).

- **Nappies.** Buy these on offer, and stock up before the birth because you'll be getting through them at an alarming rate in the early days. Check they are suitable for newborns, but maybe buy a pack of the next size up in case you give birth to a whopper. If you want environmentally friendly nappies, most supermarkets stock biodegradable versions, but they are slightly more expensive. If you decide not to use disposables at all, you'll need to buy fabric nappies, liners and some kind of bucket to put soiled liners in. See page 194.

- **Baby scissors.** Babies' fingernails can be sharp and grow quite quickly, so it's useful to have some special (round-ended) scissors to do the job. However, you should not cut your baby's nails until about four weeks after birth, as they have the skin still attached to the back of the nail, meaning you can cut the skin and cause infections. It is safer to file them with a nail file and to put mittens over them if you're worried about him scratching his face.

- **Something to bath the baby in.** You don't *need* a baby bath, and if space is tight, don't bother. You could use a washing up bowl just as successfully. If you have a bad back as a result of pregnancy or birth, though, a baby bath could be a godsend; you can buy ones on legs or one designed to fit over the top of the bath. You can get little chairs that you can use in your normal bath; these will be easier on your back because you don't need to support the baby with one arm and wash with the other. You can also buy bath beds, which is a towelling support that you lie your baby on in a normal bath.

- **Bath thermometer.** Not essential, as you can use your elbow to test the water, but if you are worried about water temperature they are quite cheap and can put your mind at rest.

- **Thermometer.** Hopefully your baby won't become ill in the coming weeks; but it is useful to buy a thermometer, if you don't already have one in your medicine cabinet, to check your baby if he does seem unwell or unduly warm. You can buy thermometers that you place under the arm or on the forehead to get a reading, but usually the digital ones that you gently insert into the ear canal are the easiest to use and give very accurate results.

- **Baby hairbrush.** Maybe wait to see if you give birth to a baby with a full head of hair, and only get one if you need one.

- **Wipes.** You are advised to stick to cotton wool and water for the first few weeks, but many new mothers can't wait to start using wipes because they are larger and easier to use. Flushable ones are now available, and if you are worried about the environment you might like to use wipes that are biodegradable. Fragrance-free wipes are best for new babies because the chemicals in the scented ones might affect your baby's skin.

- **Nappy bins.** There's something a bit yucky about putting dirty nappies in with general household waste, so it's probably a good idea to put them in a designated bin with a sealed lid. You can buy a nappy wrapper (that looks like a large thermos flask) that you store your dirty nappies in, but this can seem like just another piece of kit you don't really need. If you have a garden you can always use a nappy dustbin that you leave outside. Some councils provide designated nappy wheelie bins, which they will collect every week. They won't publicise this, so it's worth asking.

- **Nappy sacks.** You will need as many of these as you do nappies. Buy the scented variety if you are worried about less than pleasant smells impregnating your home. Alternatively you can use old carrier bags instead.

The following items are also useful but not essential:

- hooded baby towel
- baby sponge
- top and tail bowl.

Cloth nappies: what do they involve?

Cloth – or 'reusable' – nappies are an option many parents are returning to these days. The benefits are that they are better for the environment, and can save you money. What used to be an unusual and 'hippy' option is now very much the norm, easy and convenient, with many online stockists and sources of information.

Old-style cloth nappies – squares of terry fabric and plastic pants – are long gone, and modern reusables are easy, convenient, quick drying and come in a range of designs.

The first task is to decide what kind of nappies suit your family. If you don't have a tumble dryer or want to avoid using one, you need quick-drying nappies. If your baby is a heavy wetter you need high absorbency. If you're planning on using childcare, nappies that go on all in one piece are good.

You don't need to buy a full set of 25 nappies straightaway if you don't want to. It's good to get a mixture of a few different brands and figure out which nappies work best for you. In some areas you may be able to hire a trial kit from your council or local NCT branch.

As well as nappies, you will also need a nappy bucket for the dirty nappies, mesh bags to line the bucket and a wet bag for when you are out and about. Washable liners can be used to create a stay-dry layer and flushable liners can help to catch solid poo. You may also like to use a special nappy detergent to sanitise your nappies in the wash.

It's really important to read the instructions on your nappies very carefully. Most nappies need pre-washing before you use them. It's a bit like when you buy new towels – washing them makes them more absorbent. Don't use too much detergent, as this can make your nappies smell, and never use fabric softener as this will reduce absorbency.

Buying reusable nappies can cost a lot of money in the short term, but they will save you hundreds of pounds compared with using disposables, and if you look after them, they will last for years.

MUMMY SHOPPING

Probably the least glamorous part of your baby shopping, as it's quite difficult to get excited about a packet of breast pads, but there are things you need to buy for your hospital visit and to help you in the first few weeks post-birth, when shopping will be the last thing on your mind.

Something to give birth in

Your hospital will supply a gown, but you might prefer to bring in something from home. Be prepared for it not to make the journey back again, though, because it is bound to get ruined. If your partner has an old baggy T-shirt he no longer wants (don't nick his beloved Guns N' Roses tee from uni days), that's perfect, because it'll probably be big enough to give you some modesty. If you don't have anything suitable, head to somewhere cheap and cheerful such as Primark.

Maternity towels

Sometimes referred to as house bricks because of the resemblance. They tend to make normal sanitary towels look like panty liners, but they are necessary. Buy several boxes as you'll get through them quite quickly, and ensure you buy specific maternity sanitary towels, not just normal sanitary towels, as these are not as absorbent.

Big knickers

If you are normally a thong kind of gal, you're going to need to buy yourself some big pants to accommodate your maternity pads. Buy a couple of cheap multi-packs and just chuck them away a few weeks after the birth when the bleeding has subsided. Much better value, and comfier, than disposable knickers.

Nursing bras and breast pads

Try to get measured as close to your due date as possible and buy three nursing bras. Buy *one* of them in the next size up, because your breasts will swell even more when your milk comes in and you'll need a bigger bra for a bit.

Breast pads are little absorbent circles that you pop in your bra in case your breasts leak between or after feeding. They stop your bra from getting stained and save on washing.

Breast pump

If you are planning to breastfeed, it is useful to invest in a breast pump; if you plan to go back to work and want to continue breastfeeding, you can express and freeze milk that can be given in a bottle to your baby in your absence. You can also express milk and sneak off on a guilt-free date night with your partner.

Breastfeeding clothes

Many women who intend to breastfeed choose to add a few special breastfeeding or nursing tops and/or dresses to their wardrobe. Cleverly designed, they allow baby access to your boobs without exposing your whole midriff (and more) to the world, especially when feeding in public.

YOUR BABY'S NURSERY

You may be planning for your baby to sleep in the same room as you for a while, but you probably have a room in the house already earmarked as the nursery. It's worth considering if you want to plan and decorate it before the baby is born, because you may not have the time, energy or inclination after the birth. You don't need to buy much: as long as you have something for your baby to sleep in, a place to change him and somewhere to stash his clothes you'll have all the essentials.

Sleeping

According to experts, a newborn baby will spend up to 21 hours a day asleep, so it makes sense to have one or two sleep options in your home, if finances allow it. Your baby might sleep in a carrycot downstairs and a cot upstairs, or a Moses basket in the living room and a crib in the bedroom. Research the options and see what is likely to work best in your home.

Moses baskets
A Moses basket is a woven basket with handles, which most newborns sleep in for their first few weeks.

Pros

- Newborns are said to feel secure in the cocoon-like enclosed basket.

- Easy to transport your sleeping baby from one room to another.

- Inexpensive sleeping option for a newborn.

Cons

- They only last around four months because your baby will grow out of it, so it might be worth trying to borrow one (for safety reasons, you need to replace the mattress if you borrow one).

- You need to put them on a stand or the floor (not on a high surface) if you want to keep your baby close for night feeds, or want to keep an eye on your baby while he's sleeping.

What to look for

- A Moses basket should have sturdy handles.

- There should be a removable, washable liner in the basket for hygiene reasons.

- Wicker and palm are considered the best materials.

Cribs

Cribs usually last around the same amount of time as a Moses basket, ie around four months.

Pros

- Often made of wood, so they are sturdier than a woven basket.

- Many cribs have a rocking feature, which is useful when you are trying to lull your newborn to sleep.

- Good option if space is tight or if you are waiting to inherit a cot from someone else.

Cons

- Can be quite expensive.

- Have a short life of four to six months.

- Some babies don't like the rocking motion.

- If your baby is very active, a rocking crib might move too much and unsettle them.

What to look for

- Check that the crib is stable and sturdy.

- Ensure you pick the correct-fitting mattress as recommended by the manufacturer.

Bedside cots
Bedside cots, or co-sleepers, are cots that attach to your bed, so your baby is literally within arm's reach and next to you but not actually in your bed. They are increasingly popular and can be a godsend, particularly if you've had a Caesarean section, for making sure you can attend to your baby immediately during the multiple newborn night feeds, but not have to get up to get your baby from their basket or cot.

Cots *vs* cot beds
Cot beds are cots that convert to junior beds. Fans of cot beds argue that they represent better value for money, because your child can use them for longer (usually between five and eight years). The problem is that, if you have a subsequent baby, he might need the cot around the time your toddler would be transferring to a bed. So if you want to be economical, it makes sense to buy just one cot that you can use for both babies and then two single beds, because a cot bed won't last until adulthood.

Convertible cribs/cots/cot beds
Some cribs convert to cots, to cot beds, to chairs; others convert from cots, to beds, to sofas (like the Simon Horn); so there are a wealth of different options available. However, some of them can be quite expensive, so it's useful to canvass opinions from friends who already have children. It's also a good idea to look around in stores and showrooms to get a feel for what's on offer and how it will fit in your home.

Things you should know before you buy

- Your baby is only going to use the cot for two years, so don't spend a fortune on one unless you really want to.

- The Lullaby Trust (formerly the Foundation for the Study of Infant Deaths) recommends that your baby sleeps in your room for the first six months – but not in your bed. It also recommends that you **always** buy a new mattress if you accept a hand-me-down cot, crib or Moses basket.

- The slats on the sides of cots should be spaced no more than 6cm apart.

- The mattress should fit snugly and there should be a gap of no more than 4cm between the mattress and side of the cot.

- Mattresses are usually made of foam, are sprung or are made of natural fibres. Organic mattresses are gaining in favour because they are said to promote sleep, are naturally non-allergenic, and breathable.

- Cots are subject to regulations, and there are strict guidelines on safety features. Beware buying a vintage cot, however beautiful it is, because it may not conform to modern safety rules.

Buying guide checklist

- **Does it have a drop side?** If the cot has a drop side, check that you can operate it with one hand, as you'll probably have your baby in the other. Drop sides are good because you can get the baby in and out of bed easily.

- **Does it have wheels?** This is useful if you want to move it from room to room. If it does have castors at least two should be lockable.

- **Does it have an adjustable base?** Many cots have adjustable bases so you can raise and lower the height. This means, when your baby is tiny, you can put it at the highest position because it will be easier for you to lift your baby in and out, and as your baby grows and learns to sit up the base can be lowered.

- **How long will it last?** Even cots vary in size, and you might get a few more months out of a bigger one if you can fit it in the nursery.

- **Is the mattress bought separately?** This is normal, so factor in the cost of a mattress when budgeting.

- **Does it have teething rails?** Sometimes the horizontal bars at the top of the cot are coated with a non-toxic plastic coating because your baby might start gnawing everything (including his bed) once he is teething.

Bedding

Babies are at an increased risk of cot death if they get too hot at night; you should therefore aim to keep your baby's nursery at a constant temperature of 18°C (65°F). A mix of sheets and lightweight blankets or a baby sleeping bag is ideal, but make sure you tuck blankets away from your baby's face to avoid suffocation. Duvets, pillows and cot bumpers should not be used until your baby is one year old.

Sheets

Most parents find fitted bottom sheets are better because they are less fiddly to put on, but you may want to buy a mixture of fitted and flat so you can just put a sheet over your baby if the weather is very warm and they don't need a blanket.

They do tend to get quite milk-stained, so buy four of each if you don't want the washing machine to be permanently on the go. Always buy cotton because it is more breathable and easy to wash.

Blankets

Experts recommend lightweight cellular blankets (cotton blankets with an open, holey weave), because air can circulate through them and they won't make your baby so hot. We would suggest you buy two cot-size and one pram-size.

Baby sleeping bags

You need to make sure you buy the correct size for your baby (so he can't wriggle down the bag and potentially suffocate). You also need to get the correct tog rating, as there are lightweight summer ones and thicker padded versions for winter.

Baby monitor

You will need a baby monitor so that you can hear your baby if he is in his room and you're in another part of the house. You can buy very basic models that will just alert you that your baby is awake, or very sophisticated models that measure the humidity and temperature in the room; video monitors are fairly standard now, so you can even watch your baby sleep. Some act as nightlights or automatically play lullabies to your baby if he wakes; some allow you to 'talk back' to your baby if you are in a different room; some monitor your baby's breathing and movement for extra peace of mind. Make sure that you check the range of the monitor, and see if it works outside if that is important to you.

Changing table

Most people tend to change their babies in their room because you invariably need to do a nappy change after a sleep. If you are short of space, it is definitely worth considering getting a cot-top changer if there's one that co-ordinates with your cot, or if you can find one that fits the cot you have chosen.

If you have the money and the space, by all means go for a changing table unit, but bear in mind you'll only need it for a couple of years. Buy one with drawers or cupboards underneath, so that you can use it to store clothes or toys. You can also buy changing trolleys on wheels with shelves below to stack nappies and grooming products.

Finally, you can make your own changing unit by fixing battens onto the top of a chest of drawers (to hold the changing mat still and stop your baby rolling off).

Seating

For baby

For the first few weeks your baby will spend a lot of time sleeping in his bed or the pram, but if someone wants to buy you a newborn gift, a baby chair is a great idea. Get one that bounces, rocks or vibrates if you can. There's a huge range of choices out there, from the drop-dead stylish to more traditional chairs with toy bars to keep your baby entertained. These range from £10 for a simple version to over £100.

While these are really useful, do bear in mind that they have a limited life – as soon as your baby is on the move, they won't like being confined to a chair!

For mummy

If there is space in your baby's nursery, it can be useful to have a chair for you, as you might find it a nice, restful place to breastfeed. You can buy rocking chairs designed specifically for feeding and they are brilliant; they also happen to be incredibly expensive, very large and not the most beautiful of objects. You could use a vintage rocking chair or any other comfy chair (and re-upholster it if you want it to match your nursery colour scheme).

Decoration

Your baby will soon grow into an opinionated little person with his own ideas about how his bedroom should look, so don't go overboard decorating the nursery because in a few years you'll probably want to do it again. Keep it simple and, most of all, practical.

If you don't know the sex of your baby you'll probably want to keep the nursery fairly gender-neutral. Don't feel bound by the traditional baby pastel shades of pink, blue or lemon; you could go for some more quirky colours or patterned wallpaper instead.

Painting

Look back to page 111 for information about painting during pregnancy. If possible use organic paint, or look for paint with low VOCs (volatile organic compounds – solvents that get released as the paint dries). If you are painting the room, leave the stripping of the old paint to someone else. You shouldn't strip off paint if you believe that the room was painted before 1978 in case you release harmful lead particles into the room.

Wall decorations

If you want to add interest to plain walls, wall stickers are excellent because you can remove them if you get bored or want to update the room without redecorating.

You could also add interest to the walls by adding some prints or pictures. This could include a montage of family photos, an iconic children's book cover or some home-made art.

Flooring

Here are some tips on choosing the best flooring for your nursery.

- If you are putting a new carpet down, try to get it laid a couple of months before the baby is born to get rid of that new carpet smell, and the chemicals and fibres they shed.

- Don't buy an expensive carpet for the nursery because there are bound to be spills, vomits or accidents on it.

- Wooden floors can be practical but a tad unforgiving underfoot; you can warm the room up with a rug, but make sure that it has those sticky pads beneath it to stop it moving, so you don't slip.

- Vinyl flooring is gaining in popularity and you can see why: it's not only very practical, warm underfoot and easy to keep clean, but you can also get it in some really funky colours and designs.

Lighting

When thinking about lighting your nursery, consider:

- installing a dimmer switch so that you can have bright light for daytime nappy changes and dim lighting for the night feed

- when using lamps or nightlights in the nursery you'll need to keep the wires concealed, and, as your baby grows, keep the flex away from prying fingers.

Storage

Your baby's clothes will be quite small, so there's no need to get a hulking great wardrobe yet unless you want one. A chest of drawers will suffice, and you can either buy one new or paint an antique one if you prefer.

You are bound to be given lots of toys, and you can either stash them in boxes or display them on open shelves. Shelves should be securely fixed to the wall and out of reach of the cot.

Window dressing

- You need to shut out the light during daytime naps. You can buy both plain and printed roller blackout blinds.

- You can also buy blackout linings that clip onto regular curtains.

- If you are likely to travel with your baby, buy a portable blackout blind – a blackout blind that fits to any window with suction cups.

Mobiles

A mobile hanging above your baby's cot gives him something to gaze at when he is lying down. You can get sophisticated ones that attach to the cot and play music or rotate, or go for the simple hanging variety.

Remember:

- you must ensure that the mobile is properly secured, as it could be a severe hazard if it is pulled into the cot by inquisitive fingers

- black and white pictures are supposed to stimulate your baby's brain, so you might want to find a monochrome mobile or images you can stick to the wall near the cot so he can gaze at them.

9

The last few weeks

The last few weeks of pregnancy can be both an exciting and an uncomfortable time. For many women the novelty of being pregnant wears off, and they just want the waiting to be over. Even though you might be getting even more excited about finally meeting your baby, there's still a lot you can do in these last few weeks to prepare for your new arrival. In this chapter we'll take you through what you can expect to happen towards the end of your pregnancy and how to have fun preparing for your new baby.

FEEDING: BREAST OR BOTTLE?

One subject that (hopefully) you'll get a lot of information about is how to feed your baby, as it is advisable to give it some consideration before you give birth.

According to a recent survey, over 70% of women attempt to breastfeed after their baby is born, but nearly half switch to bottle feeding within a month. Many of the women who gave up said they didn't feel adequately prepared to feed their baby, and many worried that their babies were not getting enough milk, because it's impossible to know when you are breastfeeding exactly how much milk your baby has taken in.

You probably already know that breastfeeding is the best nutritional start you can give your baby, but you may feel slightly intimidated by the 'breast is best' brigade. Breastfeeding is sometimes quite difficult to get the hang of at the beginning, so it's useful to read up on it; the NHS and government have produced some very informative leaflets which you should take a look at.

Many hospitals provide antenatal breastfeeding classes in the last trimester of pregnancy; these are well worth attending, as it is important to understand how breastfeeding works and what you can do to ensure it happens smoothly. If they do not provide a class, ask for the *From Bump to Breastfeeding* DVD, as all hospitals have to provide it. You can also watch it online on www.bestbeginnings.org.uk.

The NHS has a dedicated breastfeeding helpline on 0300 100 0212, and La Leche League also provides help and advice on 0845 120 2918, so give them a call, as the solution to your problems might be simpler than you think.

Breastfeeding can be quite painful when you start: the first few sucks as your baby latches on can be wince-inducing. You might also get stomach pains, as breastfeeding stimulates the release of the hormone oxytocin, which causes the uterus to contract. Think of this as a 'good' pain, as it helps to reduce the chance of you having a haemorrhage, and it will get easier and less painful with time. The key to successful breastfeeding is skin-to-skin contact at birth until the first feed, as the smell of his mother's milk is what stimulates the baby to feed.

To help you make the best decision for you please do read up and get as much advice from health professionals and friends as you can *before* the birth. Many women are, understandably, so focused on their labour that they don't give enough thought to what will happen afterwards.

Despite valiant efforts, some women find that they can't breastfeed, and if you are one of them don't let yourself feel like a huge failure. If you are struggling with breastfeeding, do seek advice from your midwife while you are still in hospital, and your health visitor or GP should give you support when you get back home. If you're not embarrassed being topless in front of a good friend who has breastfed, she might be able to help your baby latch on properly.

Breastfeeding

Pros
For your baby

- Breast milk is completely natural; therefore, it will give your baby exactly the right amount of proteins, carbohydrates, fats and fluid that he needs.

- Breast milk is so rich in nutrients and so highly concentrated that only small volumes are needed.

- Breastfed babies are statistically less likely to have chest or ear infections, vomiting or diarrhoea, thanks to the antibodies that are passed from mother to child.

- Breastfed babies are less likely to suffer from eczema or asthma.
- As the milk is easily digested, your baby is less likely to suffer colic or constipation.
- Studies show that breastfed babies are less likely to develop high blood pressure, high cholesterol or obesity.
- There is evidence that breastfeeding reduces the chance of children getting leukaemia or diabetes.

For you

- Breast milk is free!
- Breastfeeding can help you bond with your baby.
- Breastfeeding makes it easier to travel with your baby as you don't have to worry about sterilising.
- You don't have to fumble around in the middle of the night warming bottles.
- You need to take less kit around with you if you are breastfeeding.
- Some studies have shown that breastfeeding can reduce your chances of getting breast cancer and osteoporosis.
- Breastfeeding speeds up weight loss because you use up to 1,000 calories a day fully feeding your baby.
- It's a good excuse to sit down and take it easy.

Cons

- Breast milk is less filling in the first three days before your full milk comes in, so your baby will spend longer feeding.
- It can be really hardgoing at first and make your nipples very sore.
- You can't delegate someone else to do the job in the middle of the night or have an evening off in the pub (unless you express).
- While most medication can be taken, always check with your doctor first in case it might be harmful for the baby.
- You can't start necking the vino just because you've had the baby. Alcohol is passed into your breast milk, so you are advised to keep booze to a minimum, although you can purchase alcohol-testing strips to test expressed milk.
- You also have to watch what you eat: some spicy or strong foods can affect your baby and give him wind or colic.
- You might feel embarrassed breastfeeding in public, and a recent survey showed that even nowadays prejudices about women breastfeeding in public persist.

What you'll need for breastfeeding

- Breastfeeding bras. These have clever clip fastenings that make the breast easily accessible. You'll need at least three or four, as they need washing daily.

- Make sure you have plenty of tops (and nighties) that open down the front. You can buy these really ingenious tops designed for breastfeeding that have very discreet openings and can be worn after you've weaned your child if you don't want to shell out for new clothes.

- Breast pads and muslins.

- A breast pump. You're encouraged not to use it for the first few weeks of breastfeeding to let you get your routine established, but sometimes, when your milk comes in, your breasts become so big and engorged you might have to try to express to relieve the symptoms. It is obviously useful for expressing milk if you have to go out and need someone else to feed your baby.

- Nipple cream. Your nipples can get very cracked and sore, so it's useful to have a tube of nipple cream on standby. Many midwives recommend Lansinoh, which is made from a pure form of lanolin.

Having listed all of the advantages of breastfeeding, we just have one more piece of advice: try by all means, but don't torture yourself if you can't manage.

Bottle feeding

Before every feed the bottles and teats should be sterilised (you can boil them or use a steam or microwave steriliser). To make the feed up, you should pour boiled water that has been left half an hour into the bottle and fill it up to the required level. As formula milk isn't sterile, the Department of Health recommends that you use water that is a minimum temperature of 70°C or hotter – though you'd need a sterilised thermometer to be sure of that – and only make up one feed at a time (though in practice many mothers make up several bottles at once and keep them refrigerated even though it is not recommended). Measure the formula powder using the scoop provided and drop into the boiled water, put the teat and its cover on, and shake the bottle well. Never add additional scoops to the recommended amount, as it can make your baby ill. Warm the bottle in a pan, jug or bowl of warm (not hot or boiling) water or use a bottle warmer. Using a microwave to warm formula milk is not recommended, as it can create hot spots in the milk that you can't detect (although in practice many mothers use this method).

Pros

- You can share feeding responsibilities with your partner, including getting up in the night!

- The father might bond better with the baby if he does his share of feeding.
- If you are planning on returning to work soon after the baby is born, it may be easier to leave him if he is used to a bottle already.
- Bottle-fed babies often sleep longer between feeds.
- Feeding is normally quicker.
- If you are taking medication that passes into breast milk in a way that is not safe for your baby, bottle feeding is a good choice.
- You can eat and drink whatever you like.
- Feeding in public is easier (but finding somewhere to warm your bottle is harder).

Cons

- Formula milk doesn't contain the same infection-fighting antibodies as breast milk.
- Preparing and warming bottles in the middle of the night can be a real pain.
- Cleaning and sterilising bottles can be time consuming.
- Making up bottles is something else to do, and you might become mysteriously time-poor once the baby is born.
- Formula costs money.

What you'll need for bottle feeding

- Bottles, teats and lids.
- Bottle brush and steriliser for cleaning.
- Formula milk: powdered or ready-made.

Whichever method of feeding you choose, just make sure you've done your homework in plenty of time before the birth, so that you can be fully prepared with everything you need.

YOUR ANTENATAL CARE

You'll have more frequent antenatal checks towards your due date. As a rule of thumb, you'll probably be seen at 34, 36, 38, 40 and 41 weeks, and if there are any problems with the pregnancy you might go weekly from 37 weeks. Your midwife will continue to measure your bump to check the baby is still growing as he should – if she is concerned she may refer you for a scan to check all is progressing well. She will also test your blood pressure and your urine to check for signs of pre-eclampsia.

THE BABY'S POSITION

As early as 28 weeks your baby may have turned 'head down' in preparation for birth, and as you get towards your due date, the position of your baby will become more important, as it could affect how you are going to deliver. From 36 weeks your midwife will feel your tummy to check which way your baby is facing. If your baby is breech (bottom first) or transverse (lying sideways) it is possible that a planned Caesarean section will be on the cards.

If your baby is breech at 36 weeks, you will be offered an external cephalic version (ECV). This is performed in hospital and is when the baby is manually turned from the outside to be in a head down position. This is often very successful: around 60% will turn to the head down position.

You're engaged!

Around 37 weeks (although it's often earlier for first babies) your baby's head may 'engage', which means it will drop into your pelvis in readiness for birth. This process is also known as 'lightening'. For many women it can be a relief, because it gives the ribs and lungs more space and makes breathing more comfortable. The downside is that it can feel like a really heavy weight pushing down on your pelvis/bladder and can make walking around more laboured (excuse the pun). It tends to occur later in women of African or Caribbean origin.

WHAT YOU MIGHT BE FEELING PHYSICALLY

Late pregnancy can be a joy psychologically as you know you are nearing the end, but physically it can be quite draining, as your growing bump can really put a strain on your body. We won't dwell on the bad bits, but it's useful to list a few common concerns in case they are worrying you.

- **Backache.** The sheer physical weight of your baby puts pressure on your spine, resulting in back pain and curved posture. Rest as often as you can, ditch the heels and watch your standing position.

- **Breathing difficulties.** As your uterus expands, it puts pressure on the lungs and can restrict breathing, although this normally improves once the baby has engaged.

- **Breasts.** Your boobs may already be leaking colostrum – the golden, nutrient-rich precursor to breast milk that your baby will receive for the first few days if you choose to breastfeed. If this happens, you might want to start using breast pads to soak up any leaks.

- **Indigestion.** Your digestive organs get squashed by your baby, leading to indigestion and heartburn. Try swigging Gaviscon or cold milk.

- **Insomnia.** An active baby coupled with an anxious mummy-to-be can lead to insomnia. The only really comfortable position for napping is on your side with lots of pillows propping you up. Be warned, though: when you do finally get to sleep you might have weird dreams involving the baby – most women 'give birth' at least once during sleep in pregnancy and then wake up to find, rather disappointingly, that the bump is still there.

- **Itching.** Your tummy might become itchy over your bump as the skin stretches. You can try a non-perfumed emollient aqueous cream to relieve it. In the last trimester it could also be a sign of obstetric cholestasis (see page 61), so if it occurs in areas where there are no stretch marks, let your doctor or midwife know.

- **Oedema.** Water retention is common towards the latter part of pregnancy, and your feet and hands will probably swell. If you wear rings, take them off before they get too tight; otherwise they might need to be cut off.

- **Rib pain.** Most women find that they get quite a bit of rib pain as junior gives them a swift poke to remind them of his presence.

- **Tummy pains.** Ligament pain in the stomach area is common, as the ligaments need to stretch to support the growing uterus. You might also start to experience Braxton Hicks – the practice contractions to prepare your body for labour, which feel like a tightening sensation across the tummy. If the pains get really bad or start coming at regular intervals it is possible that you have started labour, and will need to contact your midwife without delay.

- **Waddling.** Confident strides can turn into hesitant waddles, as the weight of your baby on your pelvis can make you feel like you are about to drop at any minute.

NESTING

It is perfectly natural to want to get your house in order before the baby is born; indeed, it is quite desirable, because realistically you won't get much chance after the event. However, there's a difference between doing something useful (like getting the baby's nursery ready and ensuring there's enough food in the fridge), and clearing out the loft, which is just going to make you tired and not improve your baby's life one jot.

Getting some rest and relaxation is probably the best piece of advice to help you make the most of these last few weeks, and here are some tips to help you with nesting.

- Inhaling a load of cleaning products isn't a great idea any time in pregnancy, but if the house dirt is getting you down, take yourself off for a day of pampering or have tea and cakes with a friend, and get a professional team to blitz your home. It may cost you, but it will be worth it.

- Fill the freezer. You probably won't feel much like cooking after you have the baby, but it is essential that you eat properly to keep your strength up, particularly if you are breastfeeding. Healthy ready-made meals are ideal because they just involve a quick reheat. If you are climbing the walls in boredom, by all means cook and freeze meals yourself; otherwise get them from the supermarket. If you don't want to cook, ask your partner, parents, siblings or friends if they can make meals for you.

- Do a big supermarket shop for bulky household essentials like toilet paper, kitchen roll, etc. You'll be doing lots of washing for your baby, so make sure that you buy plenty of non-biological or eco-friendly washing powder or liquid. Ecover is good but pricey, so see if your supermarket does an own-brand version. If you can't face waddling round with your trolley, shop online and get it delivered.

- Get all of your personal admin (aka paying the bills) sorted. This will probably be the last thing on your mind when you have a new baby, and if budgeting might be an issue it is beneficial to make a spreadsheet of your monthly expenditure. It's also a useful reminder to pay those bills on time. Sometimes you can even make savings if you pay by direct debit; this is good for regular bills like gas, electricity, council tax, etc. If you are worried you might get into arrears on your credit card (particularly if you have given it a pounding with baby shopping), avoid paying interest by setting up monthly repayments.

LOOKING AFTER YOURSELF

You may feel like a beached whale, but there are a few things you can do to pamper yourself and make sure you feel good during these last few weeks.

The hairy bits

It may be your idea of hell, but for some women, the idea of the amount of exposure that area is about to get means they can't think of anything but making sure everything is neat and tidy.

Women were routinely shaved before giving birth in the past, but these days it is really up to you what you do with your pubic hair before birth. There has been research done to see if being clean-shaven reduced your chance of getting an infection if you had to have an episiotomy or tore during childbirth, but a recent trial showed that it made no difference. You'll find it difficult to get near your nether regions with a great big bump in the way, so if you want to go the DIY route, you'll probably need the help of your partner to shave or trim your bikini area (get him to do your legs while he's at it). If you don't trust him, book yourself an appointment for a bikini wax a couple of weeks before your due date, and have your legs waxed at the same time.

Paint the town, and your toenails, red

During these last few weeks, why not:

- make the most of your last few weeks when it's just the two of you, and have a night out or away with your partner

- treat yourself to a pedicure: you'll probably have trouble reaching your tootsies by the end of your pregnancy, but you may still want toenails that look gorgeous

- get your hair cut. Make sure you go a couple of weeks before you are due; you can always treat yourself to a wash and blow dry nearer your due date too.

Raspberry leaf

Taking a regular dose of this herbal remedy in the last six weeks of pregnancy is said to stimulate the uterus and encourage a shorter labour. There doesn't appear to be any scientific evidence to support this view, but some women swear by it. You can either take it in a tablet form or infuse the dried leaves in boiling water to make a tea. You can buy both from a health food store.

One thing to bear in mind is that there is some evidence that raspberry leaf tea taken earlier in pregnancy causes miscarriage. Unless you are a herbalist and have specific knowledge to the contrary, stay on the safe side and do not take this herb before 34 weeks.

And relax ...

Make sure that you:

- try to get as much sleep in the bank as you can in the last few weeks. Have a rest in the afternoons if you have stopped work, and get in as many early nights as you can.

- practise the breathing techniques you have learnt for labour. They'll make you feel relaxed and more prepared for the big event.

- put your feet up and spend time reading Chapter 11 of this book; it's very important you have an idea what to do when you bring your little bundle of (wailing) joy home.

A different type of massage

One of the physical things you can do to prepare for labour is to give your perineum a massage (yes, really). The perineum is the area between the vagina and the anus, and it does come under considerable pressure when the baby crowns – some people believe that if you massage this area daily with wheatgerm oil it really helps to stretch and soften the area, and you are less likely to tear during birth. You can buy the oil from health food shops, or just use olive oil. There's a specific technique (your midwife can explain it), and obviously you'll need clean hands and short fingernails if you want to have a go.

PACKING YOUR HOSPITAL BAG

It makes sense to have your hospital bag packed and ready a few weeks before your due date, in case you are one of the 30% of mothers who give birth before their EDD. You may only be in hospital for 24 hours, but it is quite astonishing how much kit you'll need. You can break it down into three sections: labour, post-birth mummy, and baby.

Try to get it down to one weekend-sized bag, as you'll look pretty silly waddling down to the delivery room with a trolley of luggage trailing behind you. In all seriousness, space can be at a premium in some wards, so from a security standpoint it's prudent to take just one bag.

Home birth

If you're planning a home birth you don't have to pack a bag, but it's a good idea nonetheless. It's also helpful to have everything you need ready in the room where you plan to give birth. You don't want to your partner hunting round the house while you're in the middle of labour!

Things to pack for labour

- Your hospital notes and birth plan.
- Something to give birth in. (You'll be given a hospital gown, but some women prefer their own night gown or a baggy T-shirt.)
- Any medication you take regularly.
- Socks and/or slippers, as you might be encouraged to walk around to move things along. Make sure they are non-slip and expect to put them in the bin after labour. Crocs are good because you can wash them.

- Food, glorious food. Catering can be pretty hit-and-miss at the best of times in hospital, and if you give birth at night your options may be non-existent. You should pack non-perishables like crackers or cereal bars. Lollipops and chewing gum are also recommended, as you can use them during labour to focus or distract you.

- Cartons of juice and bottles of water.

- Boredom busters. Labour can be quite a long, drawn-out affair, so bring your smartphone, magazines and a good book to while away the hours.

- Smartphone (and charger). It's up to you whether you make a photographic record of the event as it happens or just the prize at the end of it, but it's a photo opportunity not to be missed. Some hospitals don't allow video footage to be taken in the delivery room, so check when you do the hospital tour.

- Music. It's probably best to go for something relaxing rather than thrash metal, but the choice is yours.

- Lip balm. Gas and air can make your lips very dry, so it's useful to keep them moisturised.

- Water spray.

- Hair elastic or hairband if you want to keep your hair tied back.

- Massage tool for when your birth partner's hands get tired. Use a cheap wooden or plastic one in case it gets lost.

- TENS machine (if you have hired one). Make sure you also take spare batteries.

What you need after you have given birth

- Basic toiletries such as a toothbrush, toothpaste, shower gel (though you can wash your vaginal area with water only), shampoo and a big towel.

- Hairbrush and make up. It sounds shallow, but there will be a lot of pictures of you with the new baby and it *may* be important to you to look your best.

- Maternity pads. Make sure they're the real ones, because ordinary sanitary towels won't cut it.

- Big, comfy knickers.

- A front-opening nightie or PJs and dressing gown.

- Clothing to change into to go home. Tracksuit bottoms are ideal: comfort is your priority.

- Your feet will probably be more swollen after the delivery than before, so take some very loose fitting footwear, but make sure you can't trip over in it.

- Nursing bra and breast pads.

What your new baby will need

- Clothes. Pack a few sleepsuits and vests, a cardi or warmer jacket, a hat and a blanket for the journey home.

- Nappies and cotton wool.

- A car seat to transport him home.

THE FINAL COUNTDOWN

- Pack your hospital bag; make sure your maternity notes and birth plan are easily at hand in a front pocket or on top of all your kit.

- Put your midwife's number/maternity unit number into your phone as well as on a separate piece of paper, and stick it somewhere where it can be clearly seen.

- Do a final practice run to the hospital a couple of weeks before D-day to get your timings. You should also check the local traffic reports on a daily basis, in case of road works or accidents that may slow your journey if you have far to go (a job for your partner or nominated driver).

- Make sure the car is working and has a full tank of petrol (another one for the driver).

- Make sure you have some essentials in the freezer. You can even freeze milk, as long as you pour a little out of the plastic bottle before you freeze it to allow for expansion.

- Ask someone to be on cat feeding/garden watering duty if your hospital stay is likely to be prolonged.

- Install the car seat and figure out how to use it, so you're not faffing around in confusion when it's time to bring the baby home.

- Charge your smartphone.

- Now relax: all that waiting and wondering is nearly over and you're finally going to meet that little person you've been growing all these months!

10

My labour

You have been pregnant for around 260 days, and finally D-day is nigh. You'll probably feel so excited you want to burst (literally) at the thought of meeting your new baby, or might be paralysed with terror about the birth. Both emotions are completely normal so don't worry!

In this chapter we look at what is likely to happen on the day you give birth. We'll take you through how to get all the information you need, what the first signs of labour might be (and what to do if you go overdue), and take you step by step through each stage of labour and the birth itself. Every birth is different, but the more informed and prepared you are for each eventuality, the better you will feel.

DO YOUR RESEARCH

While labour is undoubtedly a daunting prospect, one way to feel in control of the inevitable is to read up on it – so that when labour does come, you know very roughly what to expect, and you at least *feel* prepared. There's no escaping it: full blown labour does hurt. But we're not going to mention the pain again because you *know* it hurts – every mother you've met recently has regaled you with her birth story and, frankly, by now you're probably sick and tired of hearing about everyone else's labour. Concentrate on your own now. It won't be unbearable and you'll be just fine.

Obviously, every labour is different and hospitals have varying procedures, so our first piece of advice is to talk through the likely sequence of events with your midwife. The more aware you are of the process, the more confident you will be. Everyone has different ideas about how they would like to deliver: some go

FIRST SIGNS

If you are reading this at 38+ weeks, there is a possibility that you are in labour and you don't even know it! Your body can start gearing itself up for labour for days or even weeks (ouch!) before it finally kicks off. Those first signs can be something you didn't expect, and some women are unsure whether they're really in labour. Here are some of the first signs of labour that you should look out for.

- An increase or thickening of vaginal discharge. You'll normally have more during pregnancy anyway, but towards the end it can get very noticeable due to changes in your hormone levels.

- Backache or period-type pains.

- A show. This is when the mucus plug that seals the cervix comes away and passes out through the vagina. It often looks like a blood-streaked lump of jellied discharge – sorry, there's no nicer way to describe it. You can have a show weeks, days or hours before the onset of labour. This can be a little frightening, so if you think you have had your show, contact your midwife and she'll talk you through what, if anything, you need to do.

- Braxton Hicks. These tend to get stronger nearer your due date and can sometimes fool first-time mothers into thinking they are actually in labour. If you time them, they shouldn't be regular, but call your midwife if you are worried (or if they become regular).

- A tummy upset. Sometimes the changes that are stimulating labour can also cause loose or frequent bowel motions.

WHEN WILL MY BABY ARRIVE?

Your estimated due date

You'll have been working towards your estimated delivery or due date (EDD) from the time your midwife worked it out for you. But in all probability, your baby's birthday will be another day. Only 5% of babies arrive on the day of estimation, with over 65% arriving afterwards. So don't stress if your EDD comes and goes without so much as a twinge. In the UK we count the pregnancy to 40 weeks, whereas in France they add an extra week, and therefore a 41-week pregnancy is normal. The normal time for the baby to come is from 37 to 42 weeks, three weeks before to two weeks after the 'due date', so take your EDD as a guide and not an absolute. Easier said than done, but relax and enjoy these final days before the baby arrives.

Natural ways to get labour started

If you are keen to move things along, why not try one of the methods. They are purely anecdotal, with no medical or scientific evidence that any of them actually work, but you may have fun trying. A word of warning, though: if you have had complications in your pregnancy, steer clear of any methods to hurry things up and leave the management of your pregnancy to the professionals.

Eat me ...

Curry: It is thought that the spices in a curry have a laxative effect that may also stimulate the uterus. There's no evidence to prove the theory, though, and if you are not used to hot, spicy curries, give them a miss, because you could end up with a nasty tummy upset. If you like curry, go for it – it might do the trick.

Castor oil: Taking castor oil is an old wives' favourite which seems to be based upon bowel stimulation. As castor oil tastes absolutely revolting, there's little point in taking it – at least curry tastes good! There is also a danger that taking this could upset your stomach. Always check with your midwife before trying this.

Pineapple: This tropical fruit contains the enzyme bromelain, which is said to boost the production of prostaglandin, which softens the cervix. You'd probably have to eat plantations of the stuff for it to work, though, and you're more likely to end up with a tummy ache.

Drink me ...

Raspberry leaf tea: Some women swear by it, although it's a bit of a prenatal myth that just a cup will trigger labour. Don't drink it before 34 weeks, though, as it can be dangerous (see page 211). It's probably more helpful in preparing the uterus for birth than actually starting the proceedings off, but it doesn't taste too bad.

Touch me ...

Sex: There is some logic at work here, as semen contains prostaglandin which could get labour started. Whether you (or he) can face it is an entirely different matter. Sex may be off the cards for a few weeks (or months) after birth, so some last-minute intimacy may be just what the doctor ordered. Don't have sex if your waters have broken, you've had your show or if you have a low-lying placenta (placenta praevia), though.

Nipple tweaking: While we are on the subject of sex, there is always nipple tweaking. The stimulation of the nipple and the areola (the dark skin around the outside of the nipple) is said to release oxytocin, a hormone that could start labour. The problem is you'd need to be pretty committed to the cause, as you need to do this for one hour, three times a day, for it to work.

Reflexology/aromatherapy/homeopathy and acupuncture: Practitioners of these therapies claim that they can naturally kick-start labour. There is no scientific basis to these claims, however. If you are interested, make sure you pick a qualified therapist who has experience of pregnancy.

Stay active!

If you have the energy, a good brisk walk might jiggle your baby further down the pelvis towards your cervix; keeping upright and moving will help too.

Going over your EDD

If you are getting to around 41 weeks and there's no sign of labour, your midwife will want to keep a close eye on you, because there is an increased risk of fetal distress and a (tiny) chance of stillbirth in pregnancies that go over 42 weeks. Your midwife or doctor may perform a membrane sweep (or several over the course of the week). They do this by running a finger round the inner edge of your cervix to encourage it to start dilating. It may be pretty uncomfortable. You may experience a small bit of bleeding afterwards and a few cramps, so try not to have anything planned for the rest of the day as you might want to just go home and rest. If the sweep works, you could see labour starting imminently, or in the next few days. You'll probably be booked in for a second sweep just in case, too.

Induction

If the sweeps don't work, your doctor or midwife will probably recommend that you are induced. Many women want to avoid induction because an artificially induced labour is not 'natural'. You can't be forced to have an induction, but if your midwife recommends one, it is likely that she has the best interests of your baby at heart. If your midwife suspects any of the following, an induction will sound like a pretty good idea.

- You are approaching 42 weeks: induction means you avoid the post-42-week risks of fetal distress.

- There are signs that the placenta is not functioning properly; this could affect the oxygen supply to your baby, which could be fatal.

- Your waters have broken and there is a risk of infection.

- Your baby's growth has slowed or stopped.

- You have a medical condition such as pre-eclampsia or gestational diabetes, and your doctor thinks it would be safer for you or the baby if he made his entrance sooner rather than later.

- Your baby's movements have reduced or stopped.

One of the benefits of knowing you are going to have an induction is that you know when your baby is going to be born (unless he shows up before the induction date). We go into detail about what will happen when you have an induction on page 220.

There is some evidence that induction of labour around 40 weeks should be offered to women aged over 40 or those who conceived by IVF.

YOUR WATERS BREAKING

Sometimes the onset of labour is marked by your waters breaking, like in the movies. This is when the amniotic sac of membranes surrounding your baby bursts and the amniotic fluid inside it leaks out. It can occur without warning, which can be rather alarming. Some women describe it as a gush, others that it feels like peeing yourself, while some women only experience a little trickle.

If it is the waters in front of the baby's head that have ruptured, then there is usually a big gush of fluid which makes it obvious your waters have gone. It can, however, be the waters behind the baby's head that rupture, which means it just makes a small hole in the membranes above the head. This feels like a trickle of water. If you think this has happened put on a pad and re-check it in an hour. If it is wet, your waters have completely ruptured and you need to go to hospital to be checked out.

The fluid should be very pale in colour, or clear and stained pinkish with a little blood. It may have a slightly 'sweet' smell compared with urine. If there is green or brown in the fluid, your baby may have passed meconium (their first stool) into the uterus, and if this is the case you should call your maternity unit straightaway, as your baby may need monitoring. If there is a lot of blood, you should also put in an urgent call to the maternity unit, because it could be a sign that your placenta is detaching.

Once your waters break you should start experiencing contractions, although they may be very mild at this point. Of the 10% of women whose waters break as their first sign of labour, one in 20 of them will experience her waters breaking and labour still not starting. If this happens to you, tell your midwife: you'll probably be called in for an assessment, as there's an increased risk of infection-causing bacteria in your vagina reaching the baby once your waters have broken. Once your midwife has seen you, there are a couple of options: you may be offered an induction (see page 223), or she might recommend a 'wait and see' approach as, in nine out of 10 cases, labour starts spontaneously within 24 hours of the waters breaking early. You might be sent home and told to be vigilant in looking for signs for infection, such as a high temperature or changes in the colour and smell of the amniotic fluid. If the contractions don't start within 24 hours, an induction is likely to be recommended, as the chances of infection will continue to rise.

If your waters break very early (before 34 weeks), you may be given medication for 24–48 hours to prevent your contractions from starting. This allows time for you to have two steroid injections (see page 172) to help mature your baby's lungs and make your baby ready for delivery. You will have to be closely monitored to check you don't get an infection and may be given antibiotics. You might be given magnesium sulfate to protect the baby's brain.

It's also important to remember that the onset of labour is very rarely like you see in the movies: the vast majority of women experience a slow and steady progression of contractions and waters breaking, and for over 90% of women, contractions start before their waters break. So don't expect to have to hail a taxi and rush to the hospital before you deliver in the back seat.

THE FIRST STAGE OF LABOUR

Labour is split into three stages, called first stage, second stage and third stage. The first stage will see your labour start (sometimes slowly), and your cervix dilate to 10cm. In the second stage of labour you will give birth to your baby, and in the third stage, the placenta will be delivered. Really it's the first two stages that you need to concern yourself with the most!

The first stage is *also* split into three phases, which are described below. It covers the time from the beginning of labour, until you are ready to push (10cm dilated).

- **Early labour.** This is when your waters may break and mild contractions start. It is sometimes called the 'latent' phase and it can last for many hours, and a whole day or more is not unusual, especially for first babies. Your cervix will begin to make small changes, such as getting softer or shorter, but these may be quite subtle and difficult to detect. For some women, especially those having their second (or subsequent) baby, this phase can be very short.

- **Active labour.** This is when the contractions become stronger and more frequent, and your cervix dilates.

- **Transitional labour.** This is when your cervix is nearly fully dilated (10cm) and you are close to being ready to push and to give birth.

We'll now look at each of these three phases in turn and outline what you can expect to happen during each stage. It's useful to give you an outline of the physical things you can expect to happen to your body during labour.

Early labour

If your waters break and you start getting period-type pains, congratulations are in order: you're in labour! Inevitably your instinct is to put a call in to your midwife and say, 'I'm on my way,' but the reality is that you've probably got at least 12, if not 24, hours to go (and maybe longer). In this case you should:

- phone your partner or birth partner and get them home *now* (if only to make you cups of tea, massage your feet and time the contractions)

- if your waters have broken, phone your midwife or delivery unit to inform them and have a check-up

- if you are having a home birth, call your midwife

- resist the temptation to call anyone else; you might be in for a long wait, and there's nothing worse than the endless 'Have you had the baby yet?' stream of texts and calls. There's something rather lovely about those last few hours together, just the two of you, and a bit of peace and quiet at this stage could be just what you need.

Your cervix

The pains you are experiencing are the uterus contracting (hence the name contractions) and as the uterus contracts, the cervix – which until this point has been shut fast to keep your baby safe and sound in the uterus – starts to become thinner and open. This process is called dilation and is measured in centimetres. During early labour the cervix should go from closed to 3cm–4cm dilated and from being 2cm–3cm thick to being paper thin. It also needs to move from the back of the vagina to the front.

In a first pregnancy the cervix opens on average 0.5cm per hour; if you have had a baby before it will open about 1cm per hour or more.

How far along am I?

A word of warning at this stage: some women writhe about in agony believing birth is imminent, only to discover that they are only 3cm dilated, while other women feel only minimal discomfort and get to the same stage without blinking. Like everything in labour, every woman's experience is different. You may rush to the hospital as you're in so much pain, only to get examined by your midwife and be very disappointed about how far along you are! You may even be sent home if you are not in active or established labour yet (see page 223). In case you were wondering, your midwife doesn't use a ruler to examine you – she does it by feel.

Your contractions

In very early labour, the contractions may come every 15 minutes or so and last for around 20 seconds. The pain is like a period cramp that slowly builds, reaches a peak, then stops until the next one comes along. The sensation of proper contractions, unlike Braxton Hicks, usually starts in your lower back and progresses round to your front, although the uterus itself actually contracts from the fundus down (the top of the uterus, just under your ribcage). Your birth partner should get the hang of timing them from the point the pain diminishes until the start of the next one (use a contraction timer app). Hopefully, it shouldn't be too bad at this point – try paracetamol, a hot water bottle, your TENS machine if you hired one or a warm bath. And don't forget any breathing techniques you've learnt.

It's very difficult to describe pain, as our experience of it is subjective, but you may find you have pains in your back, your legs and obviously in your tummy. Hopefully, at this stage you will find them bearable enough to be able to walk and talk normally.

Coping

Labour can really take it out of you physically, and if you can manage something to eat and drink during this phase it's probably a good idea. Your body has a lot of work to do and it can't do it without energy; it is thought that you use as much energy running a marathon as you do giving birth, so load your body with as much energy as marathon runners do. Many women feel nauseous – either with nerves or with the pain – and can't manage to eat a thing, but it can give you a much-needed boost if you can stomach it.

If labour starts during the day, you might feel better if you stay upright and active for as long as humanly possibly under the circumstances. Maybe go for a gentle walk or potter about the house. If you want to conserve energy, watch TV, listen to music or ask your partner for a massage. You might also try a long, relaxing soak in the bath. If it starts at night try to lie down and doze, but if you are too uncomfortable to sleep, prop yourself up with pillows and watch a DVD in bed.

If you can stay as relaxed as you can during this period, you will definitely cope with the contractions better. It's easier said than done, but try to keep things as low key as possible because it's about to get a whole lot more exciting. Some women experience quite a smooth transition from early to active labour, whereas in other women it starts and stops. This shouldn't be cause for alarm but look at the checklist opposite to know when to act quickly.

Early labour SOS

If you experience any of the following, put in an urgent call to the midwife.

- Heavy bleeding. Blood from your show is normal, but heavy blood loss is not.
- If you pass green or brown fluid this could be your baby's first poo, and could be a signal he is in distress or you have an infection.
- You have a constant pain in your stomach. Contractions always come and go, so a continuous pain may need further investigation.
- You have a sudden or severe headache or visual disturbances – this could be a sign of dangerously high blood pressure or pre-eclampsia.
- Your baby starts moving frenetically or stops moving completely.

Being induced

If your labour does not start naturally, and if you are over 41 weeks, your midwife may want you to be induced. One in seven women in the UK has her labour artificially induced.

There are usually three stages of induction. Depending on your cervix and how it responds, you may need all three stages, you may be able to start at stage two, or you may be lucky and find that labour gets going on its own fairly easily – although this is relatively unusual.

Most inductions begin with having prostaglandin inserted into the vagina. This is a synthetic version of the same hormone that is released naturally in labour (and is found in semen, if you're interested!). You may be given it as a vaginal pessary or gel; this may last 24 hours, or may need to be repeated every six hours – this will depend on the formulation, but the 24-hour version is quite popular with women and midwives, as it involves fewer internal examinations! It can also be removed easily as it has a thin string like a tampon, which is handy in the unlikely event of too many contractions or fetal distress. This part of induction can occasionally take two to three days, but be reassured this does not happen often! A new cervical-ripening balloon is now being used in some units instead of prostaglandin.

Once the prostaglandin has done its trick, your cervix will be ready for the next stage of induction – that is, to break your waters. Your doctor or midwife will do this by inserting a small, plastic, hook-like instrument (similar to a crochet hook) into the vagina and making a small tear in the membranes. It is quite uncomfortable, but not particularly painful. Sometimes the waters will break on their own, and you can skip this stage and move on to the next!

After this you will need Syntocinon, which is the proprietary name for oxytocin: the hormone that triggers contractions. It will be administered via a drip in your hand or arm. The initial dose is very low, and it is slowly increased according to your contractions until they are strong and occurring every two to three minutes. Many women have an epidural when they are given Syntocinon, as it can make contractions come thick and fast. You can have an epidural when the Syntocinon is just starting (before the contractions get too painful), or you can wait and see how it goes and how you find it. The drawback with this method is that your movement is restricted, because you are connected to a piece of equipment. Your baby's heart rate will also need to be monitored electronically to make sure he is coping with the induction.

Active or established labour

As labour continues your contractions will get longer, more painful (probably) and more frequent. These contractions signify that you are moving into active stage, or established labour. Usually your cervix has already changed from 3cm thick to paper thin, and now it is ready to dilate. During this phase your cervix will dilate from 3cm or 4cm to 10cm, at which point it will be sufficiently open for you to give birth. These stronger contractions open the cervix more rapidly than in the first phase, but it could be some hours before it is fully dilated.

The contractions may be coming as frequently as every three to five minutes now, and lasting 45–60 seconds. As the contraction reaches the peak of its intensity, you will find that you need to start using your breathing techniques to 'breathe' through them, and usually you are not able to talk during one.

Once your contractions are coming every five minutes, it's advisable to give your maternity unit a call; you're probably still between six and 12 hours away from giving birth and your midwife is likely to encourage you to stay at home – as long as you can cope with the pain and have no other problems. Midwives are very experienced at taking these calls, and normally have a very good idea of how you are doing from the way you are breathing and the tone of your voice. If the pain is so bad that you need your birth partner to call for you, ensure he makes the timings of the contractions clear and tells the midwife that the pain is so bad you can't speak (she might still want a word with you, though, to check you don't just want to come in early!). Remember, you won't be in any pain between contractions!

Going into hospital

Always try to phone before you go to the hospital so that the staff know to expect you; the information they give you over the phone can be very helpful. When you arrive you will be examined, and if you are not yet in established labour you may well be sent home again – it is generally healthier and more relaxing waiting at home than in a hospital environment.

It's difficult to generalise, but normally once labour is established and contractions are coming every three to four minutes, it's time for you to pick up your bag and head for the hospital or birth centre (unless you are having a home birth, obviously).

Procedures will vary slightly depending on the type of maternity unit or centre you are going to, and you may or may not know the midwife who books you in. Here's what will probably happen.

- Your midwife will take your notes to check your antenatal history. She will ask you to confirm how many weeks pregnant you are, whether your waters have broken and how often your contractions are coming; she will then take your pulse, respiratory rate, temperature and blood pressure and check your urine.

- She will also examine your belly to work out the baby's position and listen to his heartbeat to check he's not in distress. If you are wearing

When the baby doesn't wait

One of the difficulties for a midwife trying to work out over the phone where you are in labour, or for you as a first-time mother, is that one minute you are chugging along quite nicely at five-minute intervals, and next 'whoosh!': you've had a baby. So now that we know that babies can pop out when you're not quite ready, here's a checklist on the minute chance (don't lose any precious sleep over it) that it happens to you.

- Dial the emergency number on your notes, tell them you think the baby is coming, and they will send someone to you. If you can't find the number, dial 999 and ask for an ambulance. Open the front door so they can get in quickly.
- If someone is with you, the operator might talk your birth partner through the birth stages on the phone until someone gets to you.
- If you are alone, call your partner and then call anyone you know who can be with you quickly. It doesn't have to be family: a friend or neighbour will do.
- Try to find three big clean towels: one to give birth on, one to dry the baby with and one to wrap the baby in.
- Get on all fours, put your head on your forearms and your bottom as high in the air as you can, then try to delay things by taking three short pants followed by one long blow.
- Resist the urge to push if at all possible.
- If you can't stop the urge to push and you can feel the baby 'crowning', ie coming out, squat, leaning back against a wall, so your baby can slide out and you can 'catch' him. (If someone is with you, you can stay on all fours and they can take the baby as you push him out.)
- If the cord is round the baby's neck, gently ease it over his head and wrap him in a towel to keep him warm. There might be fluid or mucus in his mouth preventing him from breathing, so quickly but gently stroke the sides of his mouth to try to shift it.
- Lay your baby across your belly with his head lower than his body to allow any remaining fluid to drain out, and firmly rub his back with the towel. Use the towel to dry him so that he doesn't get cold, then wrap him in another clean, dry towel.
- If he still doesn't seem to be breathing, dial 999 and they will take you through infant resuscitation.
- Do not attempt to cut the cord. When professional help arrives they will do that for you. Just cuddle your baby close and put him to your breast to make him feel secure.
- A short while after the birth you may experience further contractions as your body expels the placenta. This will come away still attached to the other end of the cord, and will be dealt with when help arrives.

Remember, this happens in fewer than 1% of cases, so don't worry too much.

a sanitary pad because you have had a show or your waters have broken, she may check it for signs of meconium or unusual blood loss.

- She will then probably carry out an internal examination to see how dilated your cervix is. A word of warning: these examinations can be very uncomfortable. If you really don't want an internal examination you can ask your midwife not to do one, but the downside is she then won't be able to assess accurately whether you are in labour or not.

- The midwife will start recording all the events of your labour on a form called a partogram: this is a universal graphic interpretation of the progression of your labour. If the midwife looking after you has to go off duty halfway through your labour, the succeeding midwife will be able to see exactly where you are and how you are coping from reading this chart. Many units use electronic recording now.

After 'checking in', you may go straight to a delivery room or to the antenatal ward, depending on how far your labour has progressed. Or you may be advised to go home for a while if you aren't in established labour.

Electronic monitoring

When you check in with your midwife, she will probably listen to your baby's heartbeat with a hand-held monitor. Periodically during labour, she will listen again to your baby's heartbeat. If she suspects there might be a problem, or if you have an epidural, need Syntocinon or if your labour is considered to be high risk, she might wire you up to an electronic fetal heart rate monitor. This is usually called a cardiotocogram (CTG) – 'cardio' meaning heart, 'toco' meaning contraction. You are monitored using a small machine that is attached to your stomach with elastic straps and has two sensors that monitor your baby's heart rate and contractions. Your doctor or midwife can print out the information it picks up in graph form to see how your baby is coping. Sometimes a clip (called a fetal scalp electrode) is applied to your baby's head instead of the heart rate monitor to your tummy – this is more likely if the midwife is having technical problems getting a good record, or if you have twins.

CTGs are painless, but it does mean you can't move about as much, unless you are lucky enough to be offered a wireless version. You can still sit in a chair, stand or use a beanbag, but you usually can't walk long distances. It can be disconnected if you need to go to the toilet!

In the delivery room

When you are taken to the delivery suite, you'll meet the midwife who will care for you in labour and is going to deliver your baby. While you can still function fairly normally (hopefully), this is the time to give her your birth plan and go through it, so she gets an idea of the kind of labour you want to achieve. If there are any health or religious issues that may have an impact on your labour and birth, be sure to tell her at this point. If you are pretty certain you are going to want an epidural, make that known now, too, because it may take some time to get it organised. You can usually have gas and air at this stage. See pages 172–179 for more information on pain relief options.

In some units the midwife stays with you throughout labour, but if the hospital is short of staff or has a rush on, don't be freaked out if the midwife leaves you with your birthing partner for periods of time. There will be an emergency button in your room that you can press if things suddenly speed up, or if the pain gets too much to bear and you need some relief. Sometimes it is nice to be alone with your partner for short times.

Now is the time to put all those classes and plans into action and do whatever makes you feel comfortable. If you want to stand up, squat, roll on a birthing ball or a bean bag, go for it. Alternatively you might try relaxing in a pool, having a massage or simply lying in your bed: whatever gets you through the pain. If you want to crawl around on all fours howling like a coyote, that's probably (just) OK too; one thing is for certain … your midwife has seen and heard it all before.

This is the time to take the initiative and experiment with different positions to see what works for you. Hopefully, your birth partner and midwife will be supportive and encourage you to do this, because it is *your* body and you have a right to try to create the birth that you want. You already know that gravity will give you a helping hand if you choose to stay upright during labour and birth, so if you are told you have to lie down in bed, ask why this is – there will always be a good reason, it just might not be clear to you.

This is also the time to start considering pain relief; some hospitals won't give you an epidural until you are 5cm dilated and others won't give you one once you reach 9cm, so you need to keep communicating your wishes to your midwife so you don't miss the window. Sometimes a Syntocinon drip is used to increase the frequency of your contractions if your labour slows down – this is called augmentation of labour.

Transitional labour

This is the end of the first stage of labour, before you get to the pushing stage. It starts when your cervix is around 8cm dilated, and ends when it is fully (10cm) dilated and you are ready to push. This intense phase of labour can last anything between 10 minutes and one hour. During this time, your contractions may become less frequent, but they will last longer and will be much stronger. Sometimes they 'double peak', meaning that you have one that reaches intensity, starts to fade and then peaks again.

You might be feeling sick, shaky and out of control during this phase of labour, and if you have decided to opt for a natural birth you will need to adopt your breathing and relaxation techniques to see you through it. This is where you need a supportive birth partner to reassure you. Some women find this transitional phase quite overwhelming and exhausting, but hopefully the realisation that your baby is nearly here should be the motivation to keep you going.

What you might be worrying about

- **Swearing.** Labour may be the most natural thing in the world for a woman (it doesn't feel like it at the time), but it sure isn't ladylike, and even if you never cuss or swear you might find yourself coming out with some pretty juicy expletives. The midwives will have heard it all before – and worse!

- **Losing control of your bladder and your bowels.** You will be encouraged to empty your bladder during labour, but even so there's a possibility you might leak some urine. Don't fret about it: you'll be giving birth on a huge absorbent sheet designed to mop up any leakages, and as there's going to be loss of amniotic fluid your midwife is hardly going to be able to tell the difference or care. When you feel the urge to push, it is very similar to needing a poo, and it is quite possible that you may pass a little faecal matter during birth – but that'll be the least of your worries at the time. If it does happen you won't notice: your midwife will discreetly remove it and you'll be none the wiser.

- **Being a labour monster.** Being in such acute pain can also make you very crotchety or downright rude when ordinarily you are quite lovely. It's probably worth warning your birthing partner that you may well say or do things that you wouldn't normally. You'll probably contradict yourself – from 'Rub my back' to 'Get your effing hands off me' – and may well tell them you hate them, or wish the father had never got you into this mess. All these feelings of animosity will miraculously disappear once your baby is delivered, and will only return once you become a sleep-deprived, baby-feeding monster.

THE SECOND STAGE OF LABOUR

As your baby's head moves down through the cervix towards the vagina, you might suddenly feel an intense pressure in your bottom. This is described as 'bearing down', and at this point you will undoubtedly have an overwhelming urge to push. You'll probably yell something at the midwife at this point, and she'll probably calmly tell you *not* to push as your cervix isn't quite ready. You can counter the urge to push by breathing in short puffs or panting.

Your midwife will tell you to start pushing with each contraction when she believes you are fully dilated and ready to go. Trust her guidance on this and try to follow what she says, but if you feel you need to push on your own schedule, then trust your body. You'll get the urge to push through your anus even though the baby will come out of your vagina, if that makes sense. If you have an epidural and you have no feeling in the lower part of your body, your midwife will tell you when to push. She may suggest that you wait for an hour after she has diagnosed full dilation, to allow the contractions to bring the baby's head lower. If it is your first baby, she may encourage you to push in a recumbent position as then you will be more likely to push the baby out yourself than if you are upright.

Once the first part of the baby's head appears, you can take a look at it in the mirror or feel it if you wish, or you might just think, 'Let's just get this baby out of there!'. What may strike you as weird is that once she sees the baby's head crowning, your midwife might tell you to stop pushing and pant for a bit, or take small puffs so that the baby is delivered slowly and carefully: this minimises the chance of you tearing. Also, once the head is out she may have to gently remove the cord from the baby's neck before you can push the body out.

A word of warning: for some women it is relatively straightforward to push your baby out, while for others it can be an exhausting and laborious process. It can take anything from a few minutes to an hour or more. Sometimes, despite your best efforts, you might need a little assistance.

Assisted delivery

You may need an assisted delivery if your baby is not delivering despite loads of pushing from you, or if there are signs of distress in the baby. If you have an assisted delivery, don't be surprised if you are offered one injection of antibiotics after birth as recent research shows this can reduce infections in the mother.

Ventouse
The most common method of easing your baby out is by ventouse. A ventouse is a vacuum extractor that looks like a small sink plunger. It has a plastic or metal cap that fixes to your baby's head by suction, and a vacuum pump that creates a suction effect. If you have a ventouse, you will have to lie on your back on the bed and your feet will be placed in stirrups; you will then be given a local anaesthetic if you have not had an epidural already. The ventouse will be inserted through the entrance to your vagina and placed onto the top of your baby's head. Then your baby will be 'pulled' down during contractions while you continue to push out. Usually it takes no more than three contractions once the ventouse is in position. The upside of this procedure is that you don't always have to have an episiotomy; the downside is that your baby might have a slightly pointy head when the cap is taken off, called a chignon (don't worry, he won't look like a relative of Mr Spock for long).

Forceps

Forceps are curved tongs that look like giant metal salad servers, which cradle and protect your baby's head during delivery. Years ago, babies were routinely delivered by forceps, but this is no longer the case, and forceps will only be suggested if they are felt to be the safest option for you and the baby. Forceps deliveries tend to be quicker than ventouse, so they may be used if there is a major concern about your baby's wellbeing. Forceps are also less dependent on your pushing than ventouse, so if there is still a little way to go before the baby can be born, or if you are totally exhausted, they may be preferred. The doctor will put first one side of the forceps and then the other against your baby's head, and then when the contraction comes deliver him by gently pulling – if you can help by pushing, all the better. There may be faint marks by the side of your baby's temples after a forceps delivery but they shouldn't be there for long. Your are fairly likely to need an episiotomy.

Both forceps and ventouse look like instruments of torture, but the doctor using them will know exactly what he is doing, and they will only be used if the medical team believe that your baby won't come out by himself. If you are really against the idea of an assisted birth, you have a right to question the doctor, but you will probably be prepared to undergo anything to facilitate the safe arrival of your baby.

Episiotomy

An episiotomy is a cut from the opening of your vagina into the perineum. It is never done as routine, and is only used to make space for the birth to happen or if there is a reason to speed the birth up. You're given a local anaesthetic if you haven't had an epidural, and obviously you'll need stitching up afterwards. There is a risk of infection, and it does make the healing process 'down below' rather longer than if you don't need any stitches. Most stitches heal really well and women hardly know they were ever cut.

There is a theory that women who tear naturally during vaginal births actually heal better than women who have episiotomies, although most doctors think that it is easier to do a good repair when you have been cut rather than torn. This is due to how the two events happen: with episiotomies, all the layers of skin and muscle are cut in a straight line, which is directed away from the back passage, usually to your right. With a natural tear, only the layers that are stretched to their limit are torn, often in a jagged line or in multiple places. However, this can mean you experience superficial tearing in any direction, including in the 'wrong' directions, for example high into the vagina or into your back passage (called a third degree tear, which needs to be repaired in theatre to make sure it is all working properly again). If you feel very strongly about episiotomies and would prefer to tear naturally, don't be afraid to be speak up. However, an episiotomy is only suggested when it seems safer than allowing a tear to happen, either because it will speed things up (which might be safer for your baby) or because it might reduce the chance of you having a bad tear, so you should listen carefully to why it is being offered.

How can such a big head get through such a small hole?

You may have had this thought a lot during pregnancy, and even when you are in labour, it can still be quite a terrifying prospect. If you have had an epidural you probably won't be able to feel the baby's head 'crowning', but if you haven't, be prepared for it to be very painful in the last few minutes when the head is about to be born. It's colloquially known as the 'ring of fire', but with the birth of your baby so imminent it'll be the last thing on your mind, and there's certainly no going back. Many women tear their perineum while pushing their baby out, but you should know that this is part of the normal process. You may tear any part of the skin surrounding the 'ring of fire', but it's more common to tear either the very bottom (the perineum) or the very top (near your clitoris), and about 70% of women having their first baby need stitches following birth. This isn't something to fear either, as most tears heal either on their own or after being stitched up following birth. If the tear is just skin deep, then there is no need for stitches. If it is a little deeper, then it does need stitching to allow it to heal quicker: you will be given a local anaesthetic by the midwife so you won't feel any of this, and the stitches will normally dissolve after a week or so.

Emergency Caesarean section

Sometimes your labour starts normally but you end up needing to have an emergency Caesarean section. Over 60% of Caesarean sections performed in the UK are unplanned and therefore classed as emergency, so don't worry too much if your midwife or doctor tells you that you need to have one.

There are several reasons why you might need an emergency Caesarean section, including:

- your labour isn't progressing, and your cervix isn't dilating
- your baby's heartbeat pattern becomes worrying
- despite pushing, your baby's head is not in a suitable position for an assisted delivery
- a dangerous complication has occurred, like the placenta detaching (placental abruption)
- you suddenly develop pre-eclampsia. This is uncommon, as often with pre-eclampsia you can still have a vaginal delivery, but if your baby is distressed or you are very unwell a Caesarean section may be necessary.

What will happen?

If you have a normal labour, you probably won't even catch a whiff of the obstetrician, but if they are needed, they will come quickly to assess the situation and make decisions about your care in conjunction with the midwife.

If a Caesarean section is recommended, the doctor must explain to you why this procedure is considered necessary and you will be given a consent form to sign. Speed might be of the essence here, so there won't be opportunities to seek second opinions or wait a bit longer. If the health professionals looking after you recommend an emergency Caesarean section, it is best to respect their judgement, however disappointed or frightened you might feel at the time.

Once you have consented to the operation you will be taken to theatre. Usually you will be given regional analgesis, such as an epidural, so you remain conscious but can't feel anything from the waist down; you can have your birth partner with you in the theatre. You will have a catheter put in to empty your bladder, and a cannula will be put in your hand so that fluids and pain relief can be administered as necessary.

If you have to have a general anaesthetic, your birth partner will not be able to join you. The need for a general anaesthetic is rare, but it might need to be administered if there is a need to deliver the baby immediately and there is not time to get an epidural/spinal block in place or working.

Once the anaesthetic is working effectively, a screen will be put up so that you will not be able to see the surgeon perform the operation. Encourage your birth partner to stay at the 'head' end, as you don't want him fainting at the sight of blood as they cut you open! However, if he is brave he could look over the screen to do this, as could you if you really wanted to.

A horizontal incision is made across the lower part of the abdomen at the top of the pubic bone or bikini line. It's done here because it heals quickly, with the added bonus that the scar won't show beneath your pubic hair. Very occasionally a vertical incision is necessary, but it is very rare. Next the doctors make a cut into the uterus so that they can lift the baby out. Don't be disappointed if the baby is not handed to you immediately, as he is usually quickly checked by the midwife or paediatrician first. If he is OK, hopefully he'll be placed on your chest, or given to your partner for a cuddle against his chest while they stitch you up (this could take half an hour or so, as it is a major bit of suturing).

You will usually be given antibiotics immediately before or during the operation, assessed to see if you need medication to minimise the chance of thrombosis (see page 65) in the coming days or weeks and be debriefed afterwards to explain (again) why the Caesarean section was needed and whether you are likely to be able to deliver vaginally next time – most women are, luckily.

Skin-to-skin

Early skin-to-skin contact is important, so your midwife will be keen to place the baby on your chest as soon as possible – don't worry, you won't drop him and your partner can help to steady things. Experts believe this contact is very important because it promotes bonding, calms your baby and helps get things off to a good start if you are breastfeeding. It can also stimulate hormones that will encourage the placenta to separate. Women who have their babies whisked off to special care often report that they felt a bit let down at this point, and say that they missed out on vital bonding time. If this happens to you, please try not to fret about it. Your baby will be getting the specialist help he needs to thrive, and you will bond just as well with your baby if he has to spend the first few hours, days or weeks of life in an incubator.

STRAIGHT AFTER BIRTH

Now that the baby has arrived, for the moment at least, it makes not a jot of difference whether you gave birth on a bean bag or had a Caesarean section. Ask any new mother the most amazing part of her baby's birth, and she'll probably tell you that it was the moment she heard a cry and knew that her baby was alive and well. Your partner can get involved in the process at this point, and might be asked if he would like to cut the cord (after it has been clamped). Many men really enjoy this, though some do find it terrifying, so don't worry if he doesn't seem keen.

The midwife might give your baby a bit of a clean-up, as he will be covered in blood, amniotic fluid and vernix. If there are no problems at birth, you will be given your baby straightaway. You will probably also be given the choice of having the baby delivered straight onto your tummy or dried off first. It is recommended that you have direct skin-to-skin contact with your baby as soon as possible following birth, as this helps establish bonding. If there are any concerns with your baby (as sometimes he can come out quite shocked and forget to breathe), then the midwife will check him over first, usually still in the room, and then hand your baby to you soon afterwards.

Your baby's breathing, skin colour, heart rate, muscle tone and reflex responses will all be recorded: this is known as the Apgar score, and it ranges from 0 to 10. It's a universally adopted method of assessing the health of newborns, and your midwife may well record scores at one minute and five minutes to see how he is faring. Don't concern yourself too much with the actual number – sometimes he will get a low score at one minute and an excellent one at five minutes – it just takes some babies a bit of time to 'wake up'.

The midwife will also weigh and measure the baby. You are normally told this weight in kilograms, which can be a little annoying if you only think in pounds where weight's concerned.

Baby weight

- The average weight of a newborn baby is 3.5kg (around 7.5lb).
- Full-term babies normally weigh between 2.7kg and 3.7kg (6lb–8lb).
- Full-term babies weighing less than 2.5kg (5.8lb) are considered low birth weight.
- Babies are normally between 47.5cm and 52.5cm long at birth.

A sample of the baby's blood may be taken from the umbilical cord. This could be to check for anaemia or to check acid levels if there is a concern baby is distressed.

If your Rhesus blood group is Rhesus negative and you don't know his blood group already, your baby's blood will be checked for his Rhesus group. If he is Rhesus positive you will be given an Anti D injection.

THE THIRD STAGE OF LABOUR: THE PLACENTA

It's quite weird to think that, even though you already have your baby, your labour isn't over: you still have some pushing to do! As you cuddle your baby, you may experience some more (milder) contractions as your body prepares to expel the placenta – your baby's life support system for the past nine months.

The third stage of labour, from the delivery of the baby to the delivery of the placenta, is usually a few minutes long, but can last up to 30 or even 60 minutes. Your third stage can be actively managed by having an injection of oxytocin, usually in your leg, as the baby's body is born. This shortens the length of time until the placenta arrives, reduces the chance of you having a haemorrhage from the uterus by helping it to contract, and helps to deliver the placenta.

You can also have a physiological or natural third stage, in which no medication is given. This is only advisable if your labour and delivery have been normal, you are not anaemic and your risk of haemorrhaging is low. If you want a natural delivery of the placenta, you need to note that on your birth plan and discuss it with your midwives. You might need to wait up to 60 minutes!

After she has checked your baby, your midwife may put one hand on your tummy and gently pull the placenta out with the other. It may hurt a bit, but nothing like the birth! If it doesn't come away easily or if you are bleeding more than usual, the midwife may advise further injections or emptying your bladder, or ask a doctor to assist.

When it comes out, the placenta will be the size of a small dinner plate, and your midwife will inspect it carefully to check that it came out intact and that there's nothing left inside you. In around 2% of births, the placenta does not deliver. You will need to have a small surgical procedure called 'manual removal of placenta', because if it is not removed it could lead to a haemorrhage or infection. If this happens, a doctor will come and discuss it with you and ask you to sign a consent form, your epidural will be topped up or you will be given a spinal anaesthetic (similar to an epidural, but it works more quickly) and you will nip off to theatre to get what's in there quickly removed. Very rarely a serious condition known as placenta accreta occurs during pregnancy, where the placenta grows into the uterine wall to such an extent that it cannot be detached. If this happens, you may know in advance, and your doctor will discuss your options with you before your labour and delivery.

ONCE LABOUR'S OVER

Bonding

Just a word of warning: your baby will probably not look like one of those gorgeous chubby babies from a nappy advert. Newborns invariably have misshapen heads, squinty eyes, spots and blotches (and they're pretty slimy too). Don't worry if you don't feel an instant, overwhelming rush of love for your baby. Some women say it takes time to bond with your baby; others that they didn't think he was beautiful until a few hours later. Don't worry if you feel like this. These are completely natural feelings and you're not a terrible mother!

Many women are so emotionally and physically drained after the birth that they find it quite difficult to bond in the first few days. Sometimes you just need to get home and get settled into a routine before you can really relax and enjoy your baby. Some women report that 'they can't love what they don't know,' and we respect that view. It may take time, but the unequivocal love you have for your children is like no other love you will ever experience. You will form a deep, unbreakable bond with your baby: it just might take a little time.

Alone with your baby

Once you and the baby are cleaned up (that first shower is pretty amazing), you will be taken to the postnatal ward. You might feel a bit wobbly, especially if you have had an epidural, so this is usually in a wheelchair, or on a bed if you have had a Caesarean section.

Earlier in the book we suggested that you find out what the hospital's rules are about partners staying after the birth. Many birthing centres let partners stay the night (and even have double beds to accommodate them), but it is worth finding out what the rules are, so you don't feel disappointed if he has to leave.

Most new mothers experience acute fear and anxiety in the days after birth; this is completely normal, as the weight of responsibility feels quite onerous once your baby is born. While you are still in hospital, make the most of having a midwife on tap. It can be quite an overwhelming and surreal feeling after giving birth; often you're physically exhausted but mentally buzzing. Sleep whenever you can – even a 10-minute power nap can do wonders.

BEING DISCHARGED FROM HOSPITAL

In theory you can go home as soon as six hours after giving birth, but in reality you'll probably be in for longer than that. You'll need to stay for one to two days if you have had a Caesarean section: for example, many units are now moving to a 36-hour discharge for planned Caesarean sections.

If you have had an epidural, an instrumental delivery or a Caesarean section (or some combination of these), you will probably have a catheter tube draining your urine into a bag. It will usually be removed 6 to 12 hours after delivery, sometimes longer. You will be asked to do your first wee into a jug so that it can be measured – occasionally your bladder is a bit slow to get going again, so you may need the catheter back in for a few more days.

Before you leave hospital, the midwife will ensure you and your baby are well and your baby is feeding well. An examination will be performed on the baby within 72 hours following birth, either before discharge or at home. It will be performed by a midwife or paediatrician, who will check your baby's heart, eyes and whole body. A hearing test will also be performed on the baby, either before discharge or within the first 72 hours.

All newborn babies lack vitamin K, which is needed to stop bleeding problems. Your midwife will offer this soon after delivery – it's a good idea to accept it! In some areas of the UK your baby will also be offered a BCG vaccination against TB before leaving hospital. Finally, if you don't know if you are immune to rubella, you will need to remember to talk with your GP about getting the vaccination.

Once this is all organised and both you and your baby are well, you will be discharged by the midwife. Many women need to give themselves heparin injections at home for 10 days to six weeks after delivery to stop a thrombosis forming. This will depend on issues to do with you and your baby's birth, and is a sensible precaution to make sure you stay healthy in the coming weeks.

You will probably be given some information on family planning too! You'll also get some information about your mental wellbeing, so you know what to look out for and who to get help from if you need it.

A midwife will then continue your care at home, where she will check you and the baby, as well as monitor the baby's weight and perform the Guthrie test (see page 238 for more information).

11

The first few weeks

It's a really good idea to read this chapter before you have your baby, because it's likely that you won't have much time to give it more than a cursory glance once he's born.

In this chapter we'll look at your first few days at home with your baby. This can be a very emotional and overwhelming time for a new mother, but if you follow this advice, hopefully you'll be able to treasure your first few days as a new family.

It can be quite scary when, having left the security of the hospital and expertise of the midwives behind, suddenly you are alone and completely responsible for the love and care of this little being that can't do a thing for himself.

You shouldn't feel abandoned, though: you will be under the care of the community midwife, who will be popping in on you at home for the first 10 days, and you can always call the midwives in your maternity unit. Your health visitor will be on hand once your midwife support ends as well. If you are worried that your baby is ill, you can always see your GP during the day or call NHS 111 if it is out of surgery hours.

If you are having breastfeeding problems, there should be a breastfeeding counsellor in your area, or you can call the National Breastfeeding Helpline (see page 260).

MIDWIFE VISITS

You will get a visit from the midwife the day after you have gone home; if it is a weekend, some hospitals may ask you to go to the drop-in midwives' clinic instead of a home visit. They will check your baby is feeding properly and that you are both feeling well. The midwife will then tell you when she will next visit, as it differs depending on the type of birth you have had. On average, if you have had a normal birth and there are no problems, you will have three visits from the day you go home to day 10. The baby will be weighed and have a blood Guthrie test taken on day five, and then be weighed again around day 10. The screening timeline can be seen online at www.screening.nhs.uk, which shows all the tests and checks that need to be performed following birth.

The Guthrie test involves taking a few drops of your baby's blood from his heel and placing them onto a small filter card. This blood is tested for a number of rare but important inherited conditions, all of which are less problematic if diagnosed and treated sooner. They include cystic fibrosis, phenylketonuria, hypothyroidism, sickle cell disease, MCAD (Medium chain acyl coA dehydrogenase) deficiency, and four other rare inherited metabolic diseases (see www.nhs.uk and search 'Newborn blood spot test' for more details).

YOUR EMOTIONS

Don't worry if you get what's known as the 'baby blues' after the birth of your baby: it's completely normal to feel a bit low after the excitement of your baby's birth, and for most of us it's short lived; you'll be back to your chipper self in no time (just slightly more tired).

All of your fears and stresses are completely normal. If you need help, just ask, and try to make sure that you relax and enjoy these early days.

Tips for enjoying the first few days

- Switch your phone off for a few hours a day and get some rest. You don't need to be rudely awoken from a much-needed doze by a text message pinging in your ear.

- Warn your partner that his role for the first few days after birth is that of a hotel concierge-cum-receptionist with chef and waiting duties thrown in. He'll probably spend the first week fielding calls, answering the door for flower and parcel deliveries, making cups of tea for the endless stream of visitors and rustling up your favourite banned pregnancy foods.

- Be strict about visiting times and *don't* offer to feed *anyone* except your baby.

- If you are too tired to have any visitors, family and friends who really love you will respect that decision.

- If you do need help physically or emotionally, don't be afraid to ask; friends and family are usually delighted to help.

LOOKING AFTER YOUR BABY

Now that you have another person entirely dependent on you, it can be helpful for you to have some tips and advice on caring for your newborn; these should hopefully see you through the first few weeks until you get the hang of things.

Weird but wonderful

There are some weird and rather wonderful things you should know about your newborn, so that you don't spend the first week with your midwife on speed dial.

- The first poos (called meconium) your baby will pass are dark and sticky, and are often described as looking like Marmite! After a day or so the stools become much runnier, and are yellow or green in colour if you breastfeed. Bottle-fed babies tend to have firmer, paler and smellier stools. If you breastfeed, the stools may be affected by things you are eating, so don't panic if the baby passes something very luminous. There are also sometimes 'seedy'-looking things in the poo, which are completely normal too.

- There are two soft spots on the top of a baby's head called the fontanelles, where the skull bones have yet to fuse. The skin above the front one will rise and fall (particularly when the baby gets hot). You may also worry that this part of your baby's head will get damaged, but there is a thick layer of membrane below the skin which is very difficult to penetrate (but, obviously, don't poke it).

- Babies do vomit quite a lot of milk. This is completely normal and should be a milky colour, but if it is projectile, copious or you think your baby is in pain, mention it to your midwife or health visitor.

- Babies sleep for up to 21 hours a day in the early weeks of life, but not all at once (and often only in periods of one or two hours). You should make the most of this time and try to catch a nap too.

- Your baby may be very spotty or flaky, or have rashes on his skin. It's not surprising, really, when you consider he's been hydrated by your amniotic fluid for nine months, and now he's out in the air and subjected to air conditioning, heating and so on. If you are worried about a rash, check with your midwife, but it's likely to be harmless.

- If your baby's skin is still a bit greasy, this is the remains of the vernix that protected his skin in the uterus. Don't try to wash it off because it will prevent his skin becoming dry.

- If your baby resembles a mini gorilla with lots of hair covering his body, this is the remains of the lanugo; it will drop out over the coming weeks.

- The genitals and nipples of your newborn may be swollen due to the hormones you will have passed on; if you have a little girl it's even possible she will pass a little blood into her nappy.

- The remainder of the umbilical cord stays attached to your baby's tummy for a few weeks after birth (initially he may come home with a small plastic clamp on it). It will eventually shrivel and fall off. It can become infected, so keep an eye on it and let your health visitor know if it looks sore.

- Your baby may have a squint: this is temporary while the muscles around the eyes develop.

Holding your baby

It can be quite frightening holding your new baby because he is so small, delicate and, well, *new*. The most important thing to remember is that babies have no strength in their neck muscles for the first few months, and therefore their heads will flop forward and back if you don't support them.

Remember that your baby's neck muscles may not fully support the weight of his head until around six months, so make sure that you continue to support his head and neck even after he acquires some strength in the neck muscle area.

If you have visitors over it is likely that they will want to hold your baby. Ideally they should wash their hands before they do so, and it's often useful to insist that they are sitting down before you pass your baby over – keep the head supported during the transition from one 'holder' to another. It may sound an obvious tip, but you are minimising the chances of actually dropping the baby.

Breastfeeding

You are going to spend quite a lot of time feeding your baby in the first few weeks of his life. We've already covered breastfeeding (see page 204), and must stress that how you choose to feed your baby is entirely up to you.

Even if you are committed to breastfeeding, things can conspire against you: you may have a disinterested baby or one that's not very good at sucking; you might have trouble getting your milk supply going; or your nipples might become so sore and cracked, the thought of anyone touching them makes you want to weep. But if you persevere, with the right help you will get through it and may even come to enjoy it.

You should be getting visits from your community midwife at home, and if you are struggling with breastfeeding make sure she gives you as much hands-on help as you need – and don't feel embarrassed asking for help with this.

Colostrum

For the first few days of feeding you will be giving your baby colostrum, which is the rich, creamy milk your breasts produce until your milk comes in. It is full of antibodies that protect your baby from infections and give him immunity. It is also very easy for him to digest while his digestive system gets used to working.

When your milk comes in

Your milk will normally come in around three or four days after the birth. Your breasts will suddenly feel even bigger, and may become swollen and tender. This may make any difficulties you've been having even more challenging, but stick with it and ask for as much help as you need. If you need tips on breastfeeding, try one of the helplines listed at the back of the book.

 Words from the professionals

If your breasts are really painful when your milk comes in, send out for a cabbage. Separate the cabbage into leaves and place in the fridge. Once they've cooled, place a leaf into the inside of each bra cup. Amazingly, the cooled leaves make your swollen breasts feel more comfortable – you'll need to replace them regularly as your body heat 'cooks' them, and once they are warm they no longer provide relief.

Tips for successful breastfeeding

- Are you sitting comfortably? It's important to be comfortable when feeding, so try resting your feet on a footstool and putting a pillow under your arm (or use a V pillow) so your baby is correctly positioned.

- Babies typically let you know they are hungry by turning their heads towards your breast and opening and shutting their mouths like a baby bird. If your baby seems hungry, offer him the breast whenever he wants it; it may be exhausting, but 'feeding on demand' keeps your milk supplies up. Within weeks he will be feeding quicker and be able to swallow more at a time, so feeds become faster and more spaced out. In the first two weeks it is difficult to work out a feeding routine, but this will naturally happen after the first couple of weeks, so don't worry too much about it.

- Make sure your baby gets as big a mouthful of breast as possible. You need to get the whole of the nipple and areola in his mouth; if he just nibbles at the nipple end the milk won't come out and you'll be in agony.

- If your baby is wrongly positioned or hasn't got enough of the breast in, take it out and start again. Don't just try to pull him off while he's still sucking, because it will be very painful; if you pop your little finger into the corner of his mouth, you can break the suction before repositioning him.

- Let your baby drain the whole of one breast before offering him the other. You will usually need to start the following feed with the breast you finished on, unless he was particularly hungry and drained both breasts. Some people like to put a ribbon or safety pin on their bra strap to remind them which breast to use, but it's normally pretty obvious which one is fuller and which one was drained last.

- Keep breast pads to hand. Your breasts can leak quite alarmingly; we've known women whose breasts started squirting like water pistols when they were taking a shower just after the baby was born.

- Breastfeeding can make you feel thirsty, so make sure that you keep a glass of water near you while you feed. You are also recommended to drink six to eight glasses of water a day; it might help you to keep your milk supply up and will certainly help prevent constipation. Keeping hydrated also makes you feel better physically and less tired.

- Treat yourself! It's recommended that you take on an additional 400 calories per day when you are breastfeeding so if it's getting you down a bit, spoil yourself with a big fat cream bun!

- If you are normally quite a private person, don't think you have to breastfeed in public. Request some privacy or find a quiet corner. You can also buy apron-type breastfeeding covers that you wear like a pinnie.

- Try to stick to the same drinking limits as you did in pregnancy, as the alcohol can be passed through the milk to your baby.

- You can buy special feeding tops that help you feed discreetly, as they have little flaps or openings enabling you to just pop out a boob without your whole bosom being on show. As your baby's head is usually larger than your breast, you can feed without so much as a glimpse of the nipple. If you don't want to splash out on a specific top for the purpose, try wearing a smock-type top or loose tunic that you can discreetly pop your baby underneath, but make sure it's loose enough for plenty of air to circulate to prevent suffocation.

- You'll be advised not to smoke while you are breastfeeding, as nicotine and other dangerous chemicals can be passed on to your baby.

- Take 10 micrograms of vitamin D daily while breastfeeding for the sake of your baby's bones and teeth.

Breastfeeding premature babies

Premature babies are often not ready to breastfeed immediately. Their tiny bodies are not developed enough to get the hang of the suck/swallow/breathe reflex, and this can be incredibly disheartening for new mothers. Take heart, however, because there are things you can do while you wait for this reflex to kick in.

• If your baby isn't ready to feed directly from the breast, the hospital staff will encourage you to express milk using a breast pump. They will then administer your breast milk using whatever method is appropriate for your individual baby (this will be discussed with you before they do anything).

• Expressing milk is not as effective as the sucking action of a baby's mouth and tongue. Therefore, don't get discouraged if you only produce small amounts of colostrum and breast milk with a breast pump; it's perfectly normal. Some hospitals have a milk bank so your baby can have donor breast milk if you are unable to express enough of your own breast milk.

• There is a 'let-down' hormone produced in a woman's body to assist with breastfeeding, and the production of it is stimulated by the smell, cry or touch of a newborn. As premature babies are often isolated and away from their mothers, this hormone takes time to get going. Try expressing milk as often as you can in the presence of your baby – you may be surprised at the difference in volume you can produce!

• Stress can play an important role in the production of breast milk, and parents of premature infants are under a colossal amount of it. Try to relax as much as possible and hold your baby whenever you can to stimulate production.

• Tiny babies may need a higher concentration of calories than full-term infants, so don't be concerned if hospital staff supplement your breast milk with formula. Breast milk contains on average 20kcals an ounce, but some babies need more like 22kcals an ounce, or more. Most of the time formula is added to your breast milk, but it may be given in a separate feed if necessary.

• The most important thing to remember about breastfeeding premature infants is that even if they cannot feed directly from you, you're doing the best you can for them. If you have to stop expressing milk because it's too much stress, no one will blame you. It's hard having a premie!

Moving to bottle feeding

If you choose to bottle feed, don't feel bad or think you have failed: you are no less of a mother if you give your baby formula. For more information on bottle feeding, see pages 206-207.

Hygiene is key with bottle feeding: you don't want to make your baby ill because of poor preparation or cleanliness, so ensure you sterilise properly every time, and use bottles within one hour of making it.

'Combi' feeding

Some mothers reach a happy compromise by mixing feeding, and give their babies some breast milk and some formula. It may take some perseverance, but most babies will adapt in the end, and it will be useful if you have appointments, a KIT day at work or a rare night out with the girls, because it means someone else can feed the baby.

If you want to try combined ('combi') feeding, you'll need to decide which feed of the day should be formula, and stick to it because of the supply and demand way that boobs work. Your breasts will adapt to this new regime and stop producing as much milk, so if you suddenly decide to switch back you might find it hard to up your milk production again.

It is recommended that you stick solely with breastfeeding for the first few weeks to get your milk supply established and your baby used to feeding. It is said that some babies experience 'nipple confusion' if a bottle is introduced too early and may then refuse to take the breast, so you might want to wait until you actually need someone else to feed your baby (for a night out or a KIT day, for example) before you introduce a bottle feed. Be aware that switching from breast to formula might be harder than you think; if your baby gets used to the sweet, filling breast milk, he might find formula milk much less appealing and refuse to drink it at first.

Changing your baby

You probably learnt to change a nappy in your antenatal classes, so we won't state the obvious, except to say that the reality of a wriggling baby is somewhat different than practising on a dolly!

Watch out, as some babies will be affected by a rush of cold air and pee the minute their nappy is taken off, which can be quite disconcerting when this arc of wee is heading your way. Changing nappies can be incredibly messy, so make sure you have loads of wipes and anti-bacterial spray to hand because changing mats can get awfully mucky.

Nappy changing tips

- Change your baby's nappy as soon as he does a poo, to prevent nappy rash.
- Don't let him sit in wet nappies either, as they will irritate his delicate skin.

- Clean and dry his bottom with cotton wool in the early days (alcohol-free wipes won't do any harm).

- Apply some barrier cream before you put a new nappy on.

- Some people think that your baby should have 'nappy free' time every day to give the skin a bit of an airing; if you want to do that, lay him on the floor on top of a towel and changing mat in case of accidents.

Be alert!

- Wet nappies are an indication that your baby is feeding well, and ideally he should be doing six to eight pees over a 24-hour period.

- Breastfed babies can have rather erratic bowels and may not do a poo for a couple of days. If three or more days go past and you are worried, or your baby seems in pain, seek advice from your doctor or midwife.

- Formula-fed babies are more prone to constipation, so if he's not going daily you might want to mention it to your health visitor.

Top and tailing your baby

There's no reason why you shouldn't put your baby in the bath from the word go, but if you are a little nervous you might choose to just top and tail him for the first few weeks. The best way to do this is to undress him, wrap him in a big towel to keep him warm and dip a big pad of cotton wool into a bowl of warm water. Work on the facial area first, gently wiping around the eyes, face, ears (not inside) and neck. Pay attention to the creases in the neck and under the arms, because milk tends to pool there and become 'cheese' if you don't wipe it away.

Next, wash under the arms, around the cord stump, and the hands and toes; and finally, using a fresh piece of cotton wool, clean around the nappy area – paying special attention to the folds at the top of the legs.

The crying game

Your new baby may cry for between one and three hours a day, and up to one in five babies is considered to be an 'excessive' crier when he does more than this. If your baby is crying relentlessly, it's important to eliminate what might be the cause of his distress by checking he's not hungry, too hot, too cold, needing a nappy change or poorly.

He might be hungry, in which case offer him a breast or a bottle, or it may be something as simple as needing a nappy change; he may simply be too hot or cold – touching his hands and feet will normally give you an indication of body temperature, and it might be a simple case of adding or removing a layer of clothing. If he remains warm after you have stripped him off, it is possible that he has a high temperature (the ideal body temperature is between 36.5°C and 37°C); you can check this by using a thermometer.

Do talk to your health visitor if your baby is crying constantly, because there could be an underlying medical cause that might need investigating.

If your baby is crying excessively and you have checked he's suffering from none of the above, he may have colic. One of the popular theories about colicky babies is that they cry because their immature digestive system is causing them pain; another theory is that some babies find it difficult to be 'outside' after all that time in the womb and take a couple of months to settle down. If it is colic you'll be relieved to know that things should settle down by the time your baby is three months old (although it might seem like three years when you are going through it).

Tips to relieve colic

- There are medical preparations like Infacol that you can try to relieve colic. It doesn't seem to work for every baby, but it is worth a shot.

- Alternative treatments like baby massage are said to reduce tension in the body – get a qualified therapist to show you how to do it. For more information, visit the International Association for Infant Massage (www. iaim.org.uk).

- Cranial osteopathy is a therapy that treats pain believed to be caused by the trauma of birth, by releasing tension in certain parts of the baby's body. It is gaining popularity among parents with babies who cry or refuse to settle; for more information visit www.cranial.co.uk.

Strategies to cope with crying

- If your baby is lying down, pick him up and give him a cuddle. if that doesn't work try the 'mummy jig'. All you need to do is hold your baby close to you in his favoured cuddling position and simply rock him from side to side, shifting your weight from one leg to the another.

- Sometimes a walk in the fresh air will do you *both* the world of good (keep your baby properly wrapped up, though).

- We've all read about stressed parents driving around for hours in the middle of the night trying to soothe their babies to sleep, and the car does seem to have a settling effect on some babies.

- Some babies are soothed by the sound of the vacuum cleaner or washing machine; at least you can get some housework done at the same time!

Feeling frustrated

It's completely normal to feel frustration and desperation if you have a child that cries a lot, and that, coupled with a lack of sleep, can make you feel like you are really losing the plot. If you can't bear the crying any more and there's no one around to help you, just put your baby quietly and gently in his cot, put some music on to soothe him, shut the door and go downstairs and make a cup of tea. Turn the radio or TV on loudly so you can't hear him. Then just sit and drink the tea and practise some deep breathing. It may seem cruel, but the truth is it won't do him any harm if he is left for a short period, and it will be worth it for the sake of your sanity.

(Not) sleeping like a baby

When a newborn isn't feeding he's usually sleeping – there's not much else to do at that age – but the problem is that he can't distinguish between night and day at this point, so the feeds will just continue through the night as he can't tell the difference. It's not unusual to be awoken four or more times a night by a baby wanting sustenance in the early weeks, which can be totally exhausting. The good news is that night waking does become less frequent over the coming months, and by six months many babies are sleeping through the night, or at the very least managing six hours of unbroken kip.

Safe sleeping

Twenty-five years ago parents were told to put their baby to sleep on his front, until a study showed that it was dangerous, and the 'back to sleep' campaign was launched in 1991. This campaign advocated putting babies to sleep on their backs, and has since cut the incidence of cot death by 75%. Sadly, though, 300 babies still die of cot death annually, and no one knows for certain why. The risk of cot death is highest during the first six months of your baby's life. However, there are factors that increase the risk, and steps you can take to minimise the chance of it happening to you. The Lullaby Trust can provide further information on safe sleeping at www.lullabytrust.org.uk.

Tips on putting your baby down safely

- Always put your baby to sleep on his back.
- Make up the bed from the foot of the cot so he can't wriggle down under the covers.
- Don't overdo the bedding; a sheet and a blanket should be fine.
- If he is an active baby, consider getting a baby sleeping bag for him to sleep in, but make sure it is the correct weight for the season.
- Don't over-dress him at night; just a babygro should be fine, but you can put a vest underneath if the room is very cold.

- The room should not be heated at night and should be at an even temperature of around 16°C–20°C.

- *Never* fall asleep with your baby on a chair or the sofa, in case he rolls off you and into a gap in the cushions, or cannot lift his head off your chest. Tell your partner to wake you if you nod off together – he may think you look very sweet cuddled up together and not realise the dangers.

- If you intend to share a bed with your baby, *never* do it if you are under the influence of alcohol or drugs, a smoker, unusually tired or if your baby is small or premature.

- Do not smoke near your baby, and ideally not at all, as it clings to your hair and clothes. There is a strong link between smoking and cot death, so this is the time for you and your partner to give up if you have not done so already.

- Keep your baby's cot or crib in your room for the first six months. Studies have shown that children who sleep in their parents' room for the first six months have a lower incidence of SIDS (sudden infant death syndrome, or cot death), but no one is exactly sure why.

- Sleep positioners or wedges (made of foam) were very popular a few years ago, but the Lullaby Trust no longer advises the use of these due to a higher risk of SIDS. Put your baby to sleep on a firm mattress with nothing else in the cot (such as cuddly toys or bumpers).

When to contact the doctor

During your first few weeks as a parent you will probably (and very understandably) encounter a number of times when you are worried that something is wrong; many of these things will be completely normal and nothing to worry about, but there are a few instances when you should contact your doctor. Try not to panic, but certainly contact them if:

- he is floppy and listless
- he is jittery: ie very shaky
- your baby is going longer than six hours without a feed in the first week and difficult to wake (roughly in the first week he should feed every four hours)
- all babies become a little jaundiced, but if he is very yellow and not waking for feeds
- he is crying all the time, especially if it is a high pitched cry.

Co-sleeping

Sleeping with your baby has come under scrutiny, after the science team that pioneered the 'back to sleep' research found that 50% of current cot deaths take place where a parent and child sleep together. Most of these deaths occurred when the co-sleepers were on a sofa or an armchair, but some did occur in the parental bed. In some cultures it is normal to sleep with your baby, and if you want to do it you should follow the safe sleeping guidelines on pages 243–244.

WHAT ABOUT ME?

With all this attention on the new baby, it's easy to forget that you need looking after too. You may be totally exhausted after a long labour, battle-scarred from a Caesarean section or just feel like a bomb has gone off in your (big) knickers. The birth may leave its mark on you physically and emotionally, but the good news is that time is a great healer and, however difficult the labour was, you'll soon heal and recover and be able to enjoy being a mother. We'll cover the most common body issues you may encounter post-birth and look at some of the ways you can get your body (and mind) back.

How you might be feeling

Most likely you'll be feeling battered and bruised, but give it a couple of months and any scars should have healed and bruises will have faded away (hopefully like any memory of the pain of the birth).

When the midwife comes to visit you she will not only check your baby but give you a check over as well. She'll examine your tummy to check that your uterus is returning to normal, ascertain your blood loss is not excessive, check your blood pressure and temperature, examine your legs for signs of a blood clot and look at your stitches (if you have any) to see that they're healing and there's no sign of infection. She'll also ask you if your bowel and bladder movements are OK.

Six to eight weeks after the birth you will be offered a more comprehensive post-birth check-up for you and the baby, normally conducted at your GP surgery with your doctor or practice nurse.

Afterpains

After suffering the agony of birth contractions, you'd hope that you'd have experienced the last of any stomach pains for a while, but sadly not. Your uterus has to contract back to its normal size in the days following birth (usually by day 10) and this can be painful, especially when breastfeeding, as it releases the hormone oxytocin that triggers contractions. If they are really bad, take a couple of paracetamol or try a heated pad or hot water bottle.

Bleeding

Every new mother will experience postnatal bleeding. Its medical term is lochia and it is the uterus shedding its lining of blood, mucus and tissue.

Lochia is usually very heavy and bright red in the first few days, then becomes lighter and changes from pink to brown to yellow. The sequence is quite comparable to a period, except that it lasts around six weeks instead of six days.

If it returns and is bright red again in colour or is very heavy, do tell a health professional because it could be a sign that some placenta is left inside or you have an infection. Some blood clots in lochia are normal, but if you are getting excessive amounts or the blood is smelly, again mention it because it could indicate a problem. Any clots larger than the size of a 50-pence piece should be reported immediately.

Do not try to stem the flow with tampons because they could introduce an infection into the vagina. You'll probably need maternity pads for a couple of weeks; hopefully then you'll be able to cope with sanitary towels.

Bleeding may last longer than six weeks. If it is going on for a very long time, make sure you tell your doctor.

Breasts

On day three or four after birth, the antibody-rich colostrum you've been giving your baby is replaced by breast milk. When this happens, your breasts seem to double in size and become rock hard. It's caused by a hormonal surge, and don't worry: it usually settles down after a day or so. If you are breastfeeding, you can relieve the pain and pressure by feeding your baby, but you may have to express some milk first, because they may be too full for him to latch on. You can either do this with a pump or try massaging them in a warm bath to get some milk out. If you are breastfeeding, you may also get very sore nipples, so make sure you put lots of nipple cream on them after feeds.

If you are bottle feeding, you will have to put up with a few days of pain. Try popping cold cabbage leaves into a snug-fitting, supportive bra and take some painkillers if the discomfort gets too bad. Your milk supply will dry up entirely within a few weeks.

If you get red streaky patches on your breasts and are suffering from flu-like symptoms you may have mastitis: a condition that causes the breast tissue to inflame painfully. Around 10% of breastfeeding women suffer from mastitis, which is usually due to a blocked milk duct or breast milk getting trapped in breast tissue. Although it can be incredibly painful, women with mastitis are encouraged to keep breastfeeding in the hope that they can 'unblock' the problem. Seek help from your GP or midwife, as it can lead to a breast abscess and the need for antibiotic treatment.

Bowels and bottoms

Passing a stool in the days after birth can become as fear-inducing as labour itself. If you have had stitches it's common to feel paranoid that they will burst, and the more concerned you get the less likely you are to go, so it all becomes a bit of a vicious circle and, next thing you know, you are constipated …

You probably won't burst your stitches, however much you strain, but for psychological reassurance it's a good idea to hold a maternity pad or a few sheets of tissue against them while you try to go. To get things moving, keep up your fibre intake and drink lots of water. If there's no movement in that department after a couple of days, ask your midwife to recommend a gentle laxative. It might just kick-start your system again and get you going (literally). Once you have been, make sure you wash the area where the stitches are with plain warm water. Dry very carefully with a soft towel or low-power hairdryer.

If you had a third-degree tear, where the muscle around the back passage is (partly) torn, you will have been given stool softeners automatically to make sure the stool slips out easily.

Piles after birth are very common, so even if you thought you got away with it in pregnancy you might find that the itchy little blighters make their presence known after labour, due to the pressure of the delivery on your back passage. You can buy over-the-counter creams, or if they are really bad you can get your doctor to prescribe a suppository for you. The good news is that they should go away of their own accord in a month or so.

Stomach

We all secretly hope that we are going to be the one in a million woman who just 'pings' back into shape after giving birth, but the reality is that you will look at your tummy the day after the birth and wonder if you are ever going to get into your jeans again. Don't worry if it looks saggy and wobbles alarmingly like blancmange; it's completely normal. If you were very fit before and during pregnancy, you may have stronger muscles and revert to your pre-baby shape more quickly than others; for some of us it is undoubtedly down to luck and genetics. If you have never exercised before, this is not the time to embark on a vigorous new fitness regime, but do try to get some exercise taking your baby out for a stroll. It's not advisable to do any strenuous exercise until at least six weeks after labour (ask if it's safe to start when you have your proper post-birth check-up at the doctor's). If you start too soon, before your stomach muscles have gone back to normal, you can cause a hernia.

Most new mothers are so knackered in the first few weeks that working out is the last thing on their minds, but if you want to make a tentative start on getting some strength back in your abdomen, try just gently pulling in your tummy and holding it in for a few seconds before releasing.

Once you get the all clear to start exercising, start slowly and build up; you might find it difficult to sneak off to the gym or go for a long run at the moment, so focus on things you can manage easily with your baby. Going for long walks with your baby is fantastic exercise and is good for you both: you can quicken the pace as and when you feel up to it. You can also practise stretching exercises at home while your baby naps. The key thing at the moment is to listen to your body; if you start to overdo it you might find that you get too tired. You must do your pelvic floor exercises every day.

If you have stretch marks and they are still looking 'angry', don't worry: they will fade in time. It's unlikely you'll be in a bikini for a bit, but when you do get to bare your bod, apparently fake tan can conceal them successfully.

If you have had a Caesarean section, you not only will have a big belly to contend with but a livid red scar as well. it may look quite alarming in the first few weeks, and may be sensitive and itchy as the pubic hair grows back around it. although this is annoying at the time, it is a good thing because the pubic hair will cover the scar eventually – within weeks it will start fading to pink, and within a year or two it will have faded to a thin, barely visible line. You do need to keep the area clean and dry to minimise the chance of infection. If you have had a caesarean section, you will be encouraged to do very gentle pelvic floor exercises immediately after the birth and for the first eight weeks. Because you have had a major operation, you must consult with your doctor before you embark on strenuous exercise, as you don't want to rupture your scar.

Vagina and perineum

It's pretty inevitable that you are going to feel pretty sore down below, and no wonder: have you *seen* the size of your baby's head? If you were lucky enough to get away without tearing or needing stitches, you are still going to feel quite tender and bruised for a while. Make sure you wear big comfy pants and loose trousers, and if you want to give nature a helping hand you can also try taking arnica tablets – the natural remedy that is said to boost the healing process. You can buy them from health food shops and chemists, but do check the label before you take them in case you have a condition that prevents you from using them.

If you have torn or have stitches you may need to take painkillers, and warm baths with drops of lavender and tea tree oil can help too; but don't stay in for too long, as prolonged wetting can slow the healing. If things are really bad, you can try heated or chilled gel-filled packs that you pop in your knickers, or hire a specially designed 'Valley Cushion' from the NCT or another private baby equipment company.

Stitches can be an added headache, because they itch and run the risk of getting infected. Rinse the vaginal area several times a day with cool water, particularly after going to the loo. A hand-held shower is particularly good for this; otherwise you can pour a jug of water over your bits. It's really important to make sure you dry the area extremely carefully – damp stitches heal slowly and get infected. Change your maternity pad regularly, and make sure you wash your hands thoroughly before and after.

It may sound a bit sadistic, but you really should start your pelvic floor exercises as soon as you get back from hospital. They increase blood flow to the area and can help healing. Experts recommend you do a sequence of pelvic floor exercises several times a day. If you have problems remembering to do them, use an action you do repeatedly during the day – like making a cup of tea or drinking a glass of water – as a reminder to get squeezing!

If you are unlucky enough to have a third or fourth degree tear (where the muscle around the back passage has been damaged and repaired), you will need to be reviewed by the doctors a few months after the birth to ensure it has healed well and has not damaged your bowel function. You will also be advised to start on your pelvic floor exercises immediately, and might be referred to an obstetric physiotherapist for specialist help.

Let's talk about sex

Assuming everything is healed, you will be able to have sex as soon as the lochia has stopped. If you are worried about stitches, you can wait until your six-week check-up to have them checked. You may worry that it feels 'different' down there because there may be a reduction in elasticity and you may have some raised scar tissue, but in truth most couples find these are just minor details, and things do generally get back to normal. If you have concerns that things really *aren't* right, have a chat with your GP, but bear in mind it can take months, not weeks, for everything to heal.

Don't worry if you have lost the desire to have sex in the few months after birth. You're sore, exhausted and at the moment the object of your affections is your tiny bundle of wailing joy and not the man who helped you make him. Try not to 'shut out' your partner physically and emotionally. Make sure you explain your feelings to your partner, and don't just shrug him off. You don't want him to feel rejected, and he'll understand if you explain why you feel the way you do.

When you do both feel ready to resume sex, you may find that it takes a while for you both to relax into it. You might be worried about waking the baby, you might be feeling a little self-conscious about your body if you haven't managed to shift the baby weight, or simply have a very small window of opportunity to actually do the deed, which can put pressure on you both. Your partner may feel worried that he is going to hurt you, or feel rather embarrassed about touching your breasts if you are using them for feeding as well as sexual purposes. Your breasts may start leaking during sex, which can be a huge turn off for you both; the best advice is to take it slowly and try to retain a sense of humour about the whole thing. If you discuss these issues before you get intimate they won't be half so alien or frightening.

When your midwife visits you to check on you and the baby she may also talk to you about contraception. The reason she asks is that in theory you could become pregnant as early as three weeks after giving birth (even when you are breastfeeding).

A wee problem

One thing you might not be expecting is how much it can sting when you pee after having a baby. You can alleviate the symptoms by pouring warm water over your urethra area when you urinate, and by ensuring you drink lots of fluid to dilute the concentration of your urine, which should make it sting less.

You might also feel that your control of your bladder isn't what it was pre-birth. Many women find that they leak when they cough or laugh, or find that, years after birth, they still need to get up in the middle of the night to pee; pelvic floor exercises will really help, so don't forget to do them, as it may eliminate any problems in the future.

If the problem is severe or persists once everything else has healed, do mention it to your doctor, because he can refer you to a specialist for treatment.

RECOVERING AFTER A CAESAREAN SECTION

A Caesarean section involves major abdominal surgery, so its recovery time is usually longer than for a vaginal birth. You should be over the worst after around six weeks, but some women report that they don't feel right for months, so don't worry if you don't bounce back quickly; you have to remember you are recovering from having both a baby and an operation.

Recovery from an emergency Caesarean section often takes longer than for an elective one, although that might have more to do with psychological factors than physiological ones.

Generally, if you have a Caesarean section, you can expect your recovery to go as follows.

- You will stay in hospital for 36 hours or more after the birth. With any luck you might get your own room, but not for the first day, as the midwives will need to be able to check on you regularly to make sure you are OK.

- You'll have effective painkillers while in hospital and will have to take pain relief medication home with you, too.

- Your catheter will usually be removed the next day, and the midwife will check that you pass urine normally thereafter.

- Your wound dressing will normally be removed after 24 hours.

- Your midwife will show you how to cuddle and breastfeed your baby as comfortably as possible.

- You may see a physiotherapist while you are in hospital. It is important to help you to get walking again, and to do some leg exercises to keep the circulation going to prevent the formation of blood clots or thrombosis in your leg veins. You will probably be advised to wear compression stockings, and may be asked to inject yourself with heparin on a daily basis for up to six weeks to reduce the chance of getting a thrombosis.

- Your physiotherapist will also show you techniques to laugh or cough to avoid causing problems with your incision site.

- Trapped wind is common after a Caesarean section, as your digestive system can be affected by the surgery. Sipping peppermint tea should help.

- Simple everyday tasks like walking and sitting up can be painful, so make sure that you have lots of help and support when you get home. If you are alone, make sure that a friend or relative comes to stay to help for a few weeks (or after your partner has returned to work).

- Keep the incision site clean and dry to minimise the chance of infection. Don't panic if your scar looks livid at the moment: it will shrink and fade to a pale line in time. The stitches may cause some itching until they dissolve or are removed.

- Wear loose clothing, particularly roomy pants, and avoid anything that has a band at the bikini line level, as it will press straight into the scar.

- Check your insurance policy regarding driving after a Caesarean section, as many companies insist you wait six weeks post-op before you drive. Physically you must be able to do an emergency stop, twist right around to see what's behind you, and of course wear a seat belt (which will press straight into your cut). In practice, six weeks is usually a safe time to consider starting to drive again, but make your first journey a short one and have another driver with you if you can.

- Even if you are feeling perfectly well physically, avoid carrying heavy weights or taking strenuous physical exercise until you have had the all-clear to do so from your doctor or health visitor.

When to worry about your post-birth health

There are some post-pregnancy symptoms that could signify a serious physical or mental health complication, so contact your GP or midwife if you experience any of the following:

- heavy vaginal bleeding
- fainting, dizziness or feverishness
- swelling, tenderness, or pain in your legs, especially if it is only one leg
- a severe headache that you can't shake off, particularly if it is accompanied by blurred vision or vomiting
- persistent stomach pains
- intense pain in the vaginal area
- extreme pain when urinating
- confusion, hearing voices or estrangement from your baby.

If you are really worried, call NHS 111 or ask to be taken to A&E; your baby needs you, so don't ignore signs that could indicate you have a problem.

POSTNATAL DEPRESSION AND OTHER MENTAL HEALTH ISSUES

This can be a tough subject to discuss, but needs to be covered, because up to eight out of 10 women suffer postnatal depression (PND) to some degree. No one is exactly sure what triggers it (though the drop in hormones post-birth probably is a factor) but a previous history of depression, having a sick or premature baby, recent life stresses such as a bereavement or unemployment, losing a parent when young or an unsupportive partner may all contribute.

For many women, the symptoms are fairly mild and can be accurately described as the 'baby blues', but for as many as one in five women it can be a debilitating illness.

Signs of PND

PND usually occurs within six months of the birth but may occur at any time within a year.

Symptoms include:

- feeling overwhelmed with hopelessness
- feeling too exhausted to do simple tasks
- unexplained anger or rages
- crying at the slightest things

- anxiety attacks
- sleeping badly
- inability to concentrate
- feeling incapable of making simple decisions
- feeling inadequate as a parent
- estrangement from the baby.

Looking at the list, you can guess that most of us will experience some or all of the above in the year post-birth. For most of us it'll be down to lack of sleep, but it's important that you discuss any fears or worries about your mental health with your health visitor or GP so you can get help if you need it. This is especially important if you have ever had any depression or other mental health problems before.

Baby blues usually go away after a few weeks once you have settled down into a routine and your baby is slightly less physically demanding, whereas postnatal depression lasts much longer and can be much more serious. Lots of sleep, cuddles and practical support is probably what you'll need to help you get through the baby blues. Getting out of the house helps, too; whether it's a nice walk or a night out, you do need a break from your baby occasionally. If it is more serious, you are entitled to receive medical assistance; it may be in the form of an exercise programme, psychological therapy, counselling or anti-depressants (if you are prescribed the latter, ensure you tell the doctor if you are breastfeeding as most are suitable but there are some best avoided).

Birth trauma

Occasionally women can develop severe birth trauma, which is similar to post-traumatic stress disorder and usually triggered by a difficult birth. If the birth has left you truly shaken and you feel you need to talk it through with someone, seek help from a sympathetic health professional. It is believed that discussing your birth experience can be a very positive thing to do – some hospitals even offer a birth reflections service where you can go in and get things off your chest – so if you need to share your thoughts and feelings, do speak up, as there may be help or counselling available.

Feeling scared and alone

One topic that comes up over and over when you discuss post-birth experiences is how many women feel lonely, isolated or scared once their partners have gone back to work, the midwife is no longer popping in and the only person ringing the doorbell is the postie. Undoubtedly it can be a challenging time, because suddenly you have to do everything for your baby and cope with the household stuff, and even the smallest things can be a huge deal.

You can feel like you've become quite boring, too, because your whole life revolves around your baby and you feel you've got nothing else to talk about. There are some days when it rains all day, you can't go out and you'll feel your face pressed against the front window at 6pm willing your partner to come home and take over, because frankly you have been climbing the walls. Looking after a new baby isn't all lovely walks, coffee mornings and shopping. There are days when it can feel really hard work, and here are some tips to help you get through it.

Ideas to make you feel better post-birth

- A warm bath infused with drops of lavender and tea tree oil may be just what the doctor ordered.

- If you are feeling culturally bereft, go to the movies. Many cinemas run special screenings where you can take your newborn to the latest film release on weekday mornings.

- Join a class together. There are plenty of classes for mother *and* baby, from yoga to postnatal Pilates and massage.

- Go swimming. Once your baby is 12 weeks old and has his vaccinations, you could look into mother and baby swimming classes in your area: a gentle way to start exercising and bonding with your baby.

- Go to a coffee morning. The local NCT will hold them, and even if you didn't make it to the classes, there's no reason why you can't join in after birth. You might meet some new friends and have a laugh (or a cry).

- Join an online community. Post any topic regarding pregnancy or baby care, and someone is sure to come back with helpful first-hand experience or advice; most of the big parenting websites like Made For Mums, Netmums or Mumsnet have online forums you can join.

- Treat yourself. Still in your pregnancy jeans? Sick of wearing the same stuff for what feels like forever? Go somewhere cheap and cheerful and get yourself a couple of bright tops to give your wardrobe (and you) a lift.

- Have a night out. Go out with your friends and enjoy time talking about things other than babies for a while. Or, if you are too anxious to leave your baby with anyone, take him with you. You may feel uncomfortable going somewhere formal, but babies are incredibly portable when they are tiny because they are not in a strict routine.

- Make an effort. It sounds really simple, but just doing your hair, slicking on the lippy and hauling yourself out of your trackie bottoms may psychologically do you a world of good.

My First Pregnancy top tips

You've survived none months of pregnancy, got through the birth and muddled through the first few weeks (somehow). Well done! We'll leave you with a few top tips for a happy and healthy pregnancy.

- Try to enjoy your pregnancy: it's totally amazing what you're growing in there!

- Cherish your maternity leave: it goes so fast and you'll never get that time back again.

- *Nothing* will ever beat the feeling when you gaze at your newborn for the first time.

- You don't know what love (and despair) is until you have children – but love beats the despair every time.

- Treasure each stage, because they fly by so quickly.

There will be some emotional times, some scary times, some painful times and a few moments when you wonder what you have let yourself in for, but we promise you it will all be worthwhile in the end.

Cherish the time you have before your baby is born and take lots of care of yourself. Relax and look after yourself. And enjoy getting ready to meet your baby!

Useful contacts

General information and support
Bounty parenting club: www.bounty.com
For new and expectant parents: www.babycentre.co.uk
Information on pregnancy and motherhood: www.emmasdiary.co.uk
Parents' online forum: www.netmums.com or www.mumsnet.com
National Childbirth Trust: www.nct.org.uk
    Pregnancy and birth helpline: 0300 330 0700
Royal College of Obstetricians and Gynaecologists: www.rcog.org.uk
NHS Choices: www.nhs.uk
NHS 111: 111
NHS24 (Scotland): www.nhs24.scot; 111

Alcohol and smoking
Information and advice on alcohol consumption: www.drinkaware.co.uk
Online help to quit smoking: www.nhs.uk/smokefree
Smoking Helpline: 0300 123 1044

Birth
Acupuncture: www.acupuncture.org.uk; 020 8735 0400
Aromatherapy: www.aromatherapycouncil.co.uk
Association for Improvements in the Maternity Services:
    www.aims.org.uk
Caesarean section information and support: www.caesarean.org.uk
Caesarean section procedure and mothers' rights information:
    www.csections.org
Doulas: www.doula.org.uk
Home birth: www.homebirth.org.uk
Hypnotherapy: www.hypnobirthing.co.uk; www.natalhypnotherapy.co.uk
Independent Midwives: www.imuk.org.uk; 0300 111 0105
Reflexology: www.aor.org.uk
Where to have your baby: www.which.co.uk/birth-choice

Breastfeeding
La Leche League Helpline: 0345 120 2918
National Breastfeeding Helpline: www.nationalbreastfeedinghelpline.org.uk;
    0300 100 0212
NCT breastfeeding helpline: 0300 330 0700

Childcare

National Day Nurseries Association: www.ndna.org.uk

Professional Association for Childcare and Early Years: www.pacey.org.uk

Employment

ACAS, employment relations service: www.acas.org.uk; 0300 123 1100

Department for Work and Pensions: www.dwp.gov.uk

Gov.uk, official government website: www.gov.uk

Health & Safety Executive: www.hse.gov.uk/mothers

Working Families, helps establish home and work balance:
    www.workingfamilies.org.uk; 0300 012 0312

Exercise

Guild of pregnancy and postnatal exercise instructors:
    www.postnatalexercise.co.uk

Suggested exercises: www.fitpregnancy.com/exercise/prenatal-workouts

Food safety

British Dietetic Association: www.bda.uk.com

Food Standards Agency: www.food.gov.uk

Losing a baby

Ectopic pregnancy: www.ectopic.org.uk; 020 7733 2653

Miscarriage: www.miscarriageassociation.org.uk; 01924 200799

Stillbirth: www.sands.org.uk; 0808 164 3332

Tommy's: www.tommys.org; 0800 0147 800

Medical conditions

Bumps (Best use of medicines in pregnancy):
    www.medicinesinpregnancy.org

Intrahepatic cholestasis: www.icpsupport.org

Pelvic girdle pain: www.pelvicpartnership.org.uk

Pelvic, Obstetric and Gynaecological Physiotherapy: pogp.csp.org.uk

Pre-eclampsia: action-on-pre-eclampsia.org.uk

Thrombosis: www.thrombosis-charity.org.uk

Mental health issues

Best Beginnings: www.bestbeginnings.org.uk

Maternal Mental Health Alliance: www.maternalmentalhealthalliance.org

Royal College of Psychiatrists: www.rcpsych.ac.uk

Multiple births

Twins and Multiple Birth Association: www.tamba.org.uk;
    0800 138 0509

Premature and poorly babies

Special care baby charity: www.bliss.org.uk; 0808 801 0322

Relationships

Relate: www.relate.org.uk; 0300 100 1234
The Parent Connection: www.theparentconnection.org.uk

Safety

Child Accident Prevention Trust: www.capt.org.uk
Female Genital Mutilation (FGM): www.forwarduk.org.uk
The Lullaby Trust: www.lullabytrust.org.uk
National Domestic Violence helpline: www.nationaldomesticviolence
    helpline.org.uk; 0808 2000 247

Screening and abnormalities

Antenatal testing: www.arc-uk.org)
Fetal Medicine Centre: www.fetalmedicine.com
Group B Streptococcus support: www.gbss.org.uk
Information and support for Down's syndrome parents:
    www.downs-syndrome.org.uk; 0333 1212 300

Support for lone parents

Campaigning charity: www.gingerbread.org.uk; 0808 802 0925

Bibliography

RCOG. 2018. Women with Obesity in Pregnancy. Denison F.C. et al on behalf of Royal College of Obstetricians and Gynaecologists, Greentop Guideline no.72, BJOG 2018.

Demos. 2011. The Home Front. www.demos.co.uk/publications/thehomefront

Downe S. 2009. 'The transition and the second stage of labour.' In: Fraser DM, Cooper MA. eds. Myles Textbook for Midwives. 15th ed. Edinburgh: Churchill Livingstone, 509–30

MBRRACE-UK. December 2014, December 2015, December 2016, December 2017 and December 2018. 'Saving Lives, improving Mothers' Care'

McCormick C. 2009. 'The first stage of labour: physiology and early care.' In: Fraser DM, Cooper MA. eds. Myles Textbook for Midwives. 15th ed. Edinburgh: Churchill Livingstone, 457–75

McDonald S. 2009. 'Physiology and management of the third stage of labour.' In: Fraser DM, Cooper MA. eds. Myles Textbook for Midwives. 15th ed. Edinburgh: Churchill Livingstone, 531–54

Murray I, Hassall J. 2009. 'Change and adaptation in pregnancy.' In: Fraser DM, Cooper MA. eds. Myles Textbook for Midwives. 15th ed. Edinburgh: Churchill Livingstone, 189–225

NCCWCH. 2007. Intrapartum Care: care of healthy women and their babies during childbirth. National Collaborating Centre for Women's and Children's Health, clinical guideline. London: RCOG Press. www.nice.org.uk

NICE. December 2014. 'Antenatal and postnatal mental health: clinical management and service guidance.' CG192

NICE. December 2014. 'Intrapartum care for healthy women and babies.' CG190

RCOG. 2011. Ultrasound Screening for Fetal Abnormalities. London: RCOG Press. www.rcog.org.uk

Index